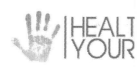 

TESTIMONIALS

"This book is a must-read for anyone who suffers from scoliosis. It gets to the heart of the connection between the mind and the body. It changed my life."

— *Christopher K.*

"If you suffer from scoliosis or just want to get healthy, you should give it a try!"

— *Julia P*

"Highly recommend this book and the exercise DVD for all scoliosis sufferers! "

— *Lisa*

"This book covers everything from nutrition, to stretching, to exercises to prevent and treat scoliosis."

— *C. Burton*

"Dr. Kevin Lau has done a fantastic job of explaining fact from fiction about scoliosis and its causes. As well as explaining modern treatment and its flaws..."

— *Mariey*

"The food ideas, stretches and core exercises are brilliant. I just started the stretches last night and couldn't believe the effectiveness these stretches did for me..."

— *Chris*

"This book has made me understand scoliosis better... Nutrition as part of the remedy to scolosis is eye opening, and has made me to evaluate my daily nutrition more carefully..."

— *Angela N.*

"This book is very insightful and offers great tips to abate some of the symptoms. It has only been a couple of weeks but we have already seen great progress!"

— *Alisha C.*

"I have had back pain for 3 years and have been to several specialists and even had a non-invasive procedure done but still had pain. I started doing the exercises a few weeks ago and I am doing much better...."

— *Norman*

Your Natural
SCOLIOSIS
TREATMENT
journal

**THE ESSENTIAL COMPANION FOR
YOUR 12 WEEKS TO A STRAIGHTER
AND STRONGER SPINE**

By

DR. KEVIN LAU

First Edition
Copyright © 2011 by Health in Your Hands Pte Ltd

Editor: Min Li

Dr Kevin Lau
302 Orchard Road #06-03,
Tong Building (Rolex Centre),
Singapore 238862.

For more information about the companion
Exercise DVD, Audiobook and ScolioTrack App for iPhone visit:

www.HIYH.info
www.ScolioTrack.com

Printed in the United States of America

ISBN: 9810770979
EAN-13: 978-981-07-7097-6

DISCLAIMER

What information and material is found in this book is purely for educational purposes only and is in no way intended to be used for diagnosis, treatment, or prevention of any conditions; it is not intended to replace necessary professional medical treatments and evaluations. Any consequences from the use of any material contained in this book and associated material rest totally with the individual; the author, editor, and publisher of these materials bears no responsibility for any injury, loss, or damages associated with this program. Use at your own risk and under your own judgment. Any individual with pre-existing conditions or known health concerns are strongly urged to contact professional, medical help in diagnosing, evaluating, and treating said conditions. Use of this program should be in conjunction with any prescribed treatments and should be approved by your doctor or health care provider prior to starting.

TABLE OF CONTENTS

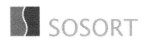

SOSORT

INTERNATIONAL *SOCIETY ON SCOLIOSIS ORTHOPAEDIC AND REHABILITATION TREATMENT*

In recognition of his contributions to the care and conservative treatment of scoliosis

Kevin LAU, DC

Singapore, Singapore

is hereby declared
Associate Member of **SOSORT** *in 2012*

Stefano Negrini, MD, Italy
President

Patrick Knott, PhD, PA-C
General Secretary

ΛCΛ American Chiropractic Association

THE AMERICAN CHIROPRACTIC ASSOCIATION IS PLEASED TO GRANT THIS CERTIFICATE OF MEMBERSHIP TO

Kevin Lau, D.C.

I HEREBY CERTIFY THAT THIS DOCTOR OF CHIROPRACTIC IS A MEMBER OF THE AMERICAN CHIROPRACTIC ASSOCIATION, WHICH SUPPORTS PATIENTS' RIGHTS AND PATIENT TREATMENT REIMBURSEMENT, AND HAS PLEDGED TO ABIDE BY THE ACA CODE OF ETHICS, WHICH IS BASED UPON THE FUNDAMENTAL PRINCIPLE THAT THE PARAMOUNT PURPOSE OF THE CHIROPRACTOR'S PROFESSIONAL SERVICES SHALL BE TO BENEFIT THE PATIENT.

Keith S. Overland, DC
President

April 17, 2012
Date

ACA's PURPOSE
To provide leadership in health care and a positive vision for the chiropractic profession and it. 7 natural approach to health and wellness

ACA's MISSION
To preserve, protect, improve and promote the chiropractic profession and the services of Doctors of Chiropractic for the benefit of patients they serve

ACA's VISION
To transform health care from a focus on disease to a focus on wellness

---

Dr Kevin Lau is a graduate in Doctor of Chiropractic from RMIT University in Melbourne Australia and Masters in Holistic Nutrition from Clayton College of Natural Health in USA. He is a member of International Society On Scoliosis Orthopaedic and Rehabilitation Treatment (SOSORT), the leading international society on conservative treatment of spinal deformities.

Acknowledgments

This book is dedicated to my loving family, my true friends, and my patients, whose love, support, and inspiration have helped me form a better understanding of the best ways to care for the spine and for helping me to understand the breakthrough discoveries that are being made.

Additional Thanks and Credits

I would also like to thank the doctors, scientist, clinical technicians, patients, and individuals who have had a part in this book, either through information passed on to me or through their inspiring stories of bravery and success. Thank you.

PART 1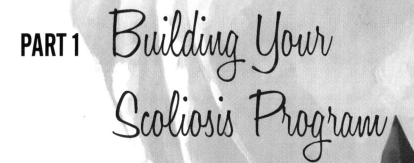

Building Your
Scoliosis Program

Chapter 1

Introduction

Sarah was an active young girl who turned 13 in 2007. Her growth and development has always been great and at the age of 13, she has managed to grow a little taller than her mother who was 5'3.

Sarah was active in sports and had a fairly dynamic routine when she gradually developed mild backache. Attributing it to her sports related activities, neither Sarah not her parents paid any special attention. Apart from occasional feeling of fatigue, Sarah didn't really develop any distinguishable symptoms or signs,

This would have continued even further until one day Sarah's mother noticed something while changing her clothes. She noticed a pretty distinguishable asymmetry in her back-region. Having seen Sarah's grandmother going through the similar symptoms, Sarah's mother had to no difficulty in analyzing the situation that her little daughter has developed Scoliosis.

Unfortunately, scoliosis is slow to develop and by the time most people realize, disease is already in advanced stages.

Luckily, the mother of Sarah was concerned who got her help just in the right time. I still remember when Sarah's mother contacted me at my clinic, she was visible upset.

I suggested Sarah to perform some exercises and in case, her symptoms did not reverse, she may have to undergo surgery.

Sarah's parents were really concerned thinking about the future outcome and her overall health. They shared all their queries and questions with me and those are the same questions who many of you have, while going through scoliosis management.

- Would she ever be able to feel fine again?

- Would she be able to get rid of these embarrassing and discomforting braces?

- Would she ever be able to live a normal life again?

- Is there a solution outside of surgery?

If all these questions have been troubling you; here is a sign if relief. The answer to all the above questions is a YES, with a BIG IF!!!

But before determining the Ifs of scoliosis management; here is a checklist to see where you stand right now?

Scoliosis may be asymptomatic (i.e. only sub- clinical) but it can also present with:

- Moderate to severe backache that may be disabling and affect the quality of life

- Classic and noticeable physical disfigurement that puts your confidence, self- courage and presentation at stake.

- Psychological and emotional disorders that follow the scoliosis and may range from mood disorders to severe depression.

- Impairment of nerve dysfunction as a result of moderate to severe nerve damage as a result of degeneration of intervertebral discs.

You may be experiencing most of these symptoms and all those who are not experiencing any of the symptoms; here is a bad news!

You are at the verge of developing these symptoms at any point of your life!

Isn't it distressing? At this point you have any of the three routes!

- Don't do anything and always live in the fear of developing these symptoms of living with these symptoms

- Adopt medical or interventive therapy like braces and wait until the braces play its role

- Go for surgical therapy and fight with all complications pertinent to surgery..

Oh but wait a minute, instead of waiting for medical or surgical procedure to take its course; isn't it a better idea to play your own role and work for your own body.

Being a nutritionist, chiropractor and strong believer of holistic methods of treatment; I strongly recommend to give your body a chance and little support to fight scoliosis.

I know most people are afraid to take the chance and practice alternative treatment for a condition as scary as SCOLIOSIS; but I assure you, your body has immense potential and if you get a chance to study my books on scoliosis; you will realize that the development of scoliosis is a failure of your immune system because of the undue stress and strain that your body have to go through because of your slackness and unnatural living methods.

In this workbook, I will start from the beginning and no matter where you stand in terms of your nutritional status and physical stability; IF you follow the guidelines in this workbook, you will achieve health, well- being and prosperity. This is not only limited to scoliosis but in terms of all the standards.

What you may need to do?

In order to get rid of braces, live a comfortable life free of agony and distress without any surgery; you don't have to spend hundreds of dollars; you don't have to lose kilos of weight and you don't have to undergo any hassle. Isn't it too good to be true?

It sure is--- That is what we call holistic or natural method of living.

An Overview of Paleo Diets for Scoliosis

Diet or nutrition is the most important and integral force that holds your body together. I am not expecting you to waste any amount of money in buying medications, drugs or supplements; this is because natural diet supplies medications and nutrients without needing supplementation.

Paleo diet is I believe the best solution to all your problems (not limited to scoliosis alone). The current trend of diseases and metabolic disorders suggest that the ancient caveman were far healthy and nutritionally prosperous than what are today; despite the fact that we are more advanced scientifically and knows more about diseases; we are living an unhealthy and vulnerable life.

Having said all this; Research indicates that scoliosis has partially genetic origin. Your genes are what make you special and unique. This indicates that some times we consume nutrients that are not well- suited by our body or by our genes (for example any time you try out a new cuisine; you are metabolically challenging your body). You may have an idea that over the time, we have travelled far from our roots and original form of nutrition.

Fast food, junk food, processed and refined food are not our natural and original form of nutrition; however, if you still try to consume it for longer period of time; you should keep yourself prepared mentally and physically for a metabolic change. We all have different capacities to bear environmental or metabolic changes; for example when you travel not all of you develops motion sickness or after eating from a cart, not all of you develop diarrhea.

In my first book "Your Plan for Natural Scoliosis Prevention and Treatment", I emphasized on the importance of maintaining a natural and organic diet that contains all the rich nutrients.

Eating Paleo diet according to your metabolic type will effectively help you to work with your genes and help you in the maintaining and regaining your nutritional as well as biochemical balance. Paleo diet also supports your muscles, healthy bones and optimal immune function. In the end you will find it's not only a diet, but also a lifestyle, that will slowly and gradually improve your physical, mental and psychological health.

An Overview of Corrective Exercises for Scoliosis

In part 3 of my first book, I introduced body balancing stretches, core stability exercises and body alignment exercises. I strongly suggest you to start working on these exercises. There are a number of benefits that may follow if you continue the exercise regimen religiously.

A few potential benefits that are reported by my patients include:

- Improvement in the curvature of spine and tremendous improvement in the quality of systemic functioning.

- Untiring energy levels that keeps you active; physically, mentally and psychologically.

- Improvement in overall health.

- Persistent improvement in the quality of symptoms.

- You feel have tremendous and unbeatable energy levels that keeps you going all day long and decrease the rate of degeneration in other parts of your body.

There is one thing about scoliosis that a lot of people tend to ignore. Scoliosis develop because of your body not being able to keep up with the aging process, poor environmental set up, physical damage. Are you aware that any persistent pressure or strain on spine can increase the risk of immune mediated damage?

Yes, indeed it does- but the good news is, you can get rid of all the ailments with proper exercise and physical activity.

Why is this Journal Important to My Recovery?

I emphasize on the need of having a work-book when you are working on holistic health program because:

- Unlike medications and surgical procedures; holistic methods of care is a lifestyle that you have to incorporate for the rest of your life. You may not get a chance to see a practitioner every now and then and you may not see the results the very next day; but I assure you if you keep a record, you will realize how well are you improving.

- Don't you find it amazing that once you try to treat your muscular pain issues or aches by medications, how disease shift from bones to involve your kidneys and liver also?

Obviously, this is not what you want to do with your body. Its more like spreading the disease from one part to all parts of your body; however, once you start following this work-book, you will realize that mere modifications in your diet and physical activities can improve the health of all your systems.

I am sure those of you who are suffering from constant nagging pain and discomfort often wonder why US?

It is pretty simple, you will realize after following this work-book that throughout our body, we have a few trigger points. (I will guide you how to mark those trigger spots in this work-book).

Upon stimulation, these trigger spots send pain signals to different parts of your body according to the distribution of pain receptors and rely-stations. If you don't take charge of your body and this overt stimulation is not stopped, your muscles may weaken over time and become less capable of supporting your body and tissues. The repeated and ongoing inflammatory process can make your body lose flexibility and strength, resulting in further deterioration and permanent damage to neural and musculo-skeletal system.

I just want you to experience the power of holistic care and maintain your compliance towards a healthier way of living. To help ease your learning, I have also worked on a companion exercise DVD for visual demonstration. With this work-book, you can actually keep a record of your progress that will increase the success rate of overall therapy and maintain your compliance and interest in the program by serving as a constant source of motivation.

Chapter 2

Instruction

Tips for using this workbook

Most of the time people think they know about balanced nutrition and types of foods that are healthy for their body; when they don't. My aim is to make you more oriented towards identifying your actual metabolic type. This is required so that you can give your body what it needs (and not what your craving demands).

This workbook will enable you to maintain a track record of your daily dietary intake and exercise for 12 weeks. 12 weeks because this period is enough to:

- Re-program your genes

- Learn what your body needs

- Getting your system and metabolism in track

- Detoxification of your body to eliminate the toxins ad inflammatory mediators that are affecting your systemic sanctuary.

- Getting back the hormonal control of your body.

I am sure, after recording your comments after consuming the foods under paleo recommendations, you will learn your metabolic type in a few weeks. Similarly, not all the exercises or body movements are for everyone. Learning where your natural powers area and working with your muscles (instead of opposing natural posture) will prevent the recurrence of scoliosis and other degenerative issues.

I have tried to keep everything extremely simple and objective. Natural and organic lifestyle will enable you to re-program your genes to get them involved in the path to rehabilitation. I wish you all the best in your journey to better health and a stronger spine within a few months.

The only aim of indulging you in using this work-book is to maintain your compliance. Without proper and inadequate motivation and positive-feedback, it is very difficult to maintain your compliance for longer period of time.

What this work book will demand from you?

The aim of this workbook is to keep all your efforts in achieving optimal health fully organized and focused. It will enable you to record your diet, your daily exercise pattern and improvements in your health with therapy.

In order to get maximally benefitted from the holistic methods of care and achieving perfect health without any surgical, medical or pharmacological intervention here is what you have to do.

What to expect in the book:

This workbook contains all the questionaires, tables, diagrams and worksheets that you need to complete your scoliosis program.

1. METABOLIC TYPING CHALLENGE

This simple interview styled questionaire is to be completed at the beginning of your program to determine your metabolic type.

How to use:

Identify your metabolic type by your honest responses to every given question in "Metabolic Typing Challenge" on page 74.

It is the first step to find out tailor-made foods for your unique body based on paleo stance. The requirements and demands of every individual are different and knowing your metabolic type can ease the process of delivering the nutrients that your body demands.

	Metabolic Typing Challenge		
✓	ANSWER #1	***DIET QUERY*** ✓	ANSWER #2
		APPETITE (In general)	
		DESSERTS	
		EATING BEFORE BED	
		EATING HABITS	
		4 HOURS+ WITHOUT EATING	
		ORANGE JUICE ALONE	
		SKIPPING MEALS	
		SNACKING	
		DIET SECTION TOTALS	
✓	ANSWER #1	***PHYSICAL QUERY*** ✓	ANSWER #2
		BUILD	
		DIGESTION (What is your tendency?)	
		EAR COLOUR	
		EYES – PUPIL SIZE	
		HANDS – TEMPERATURE	
		LIGHT – STRONG, BRIGHT	
		SKIN – FACIAL COMPLEXION	
		SKIN – INSECT BITES/STINGS	
		PHYSICAL SECTION TOTALS	

✓	ANSWER #1	***PSYCH QUERY***	✓	ANSWER #2
		ACHIEVEMENT		
		ACTIVITY LEVEL		
		ANGER		
		ARISING/RETIRING TIME (toward, without alarm clock)		
		CLIMATE PREFERENCE		
		COMPETITIVE		
		ENDURANCE		
		EXPRESSION OF THOUGHT		
		EXERCISE		
		IMPATIENT		
		ORGANIZATION		
		PERFECTION		
		PERSONAL STANDARD		
		PERSONALITY		
		PRODUCTIVE		
		SOCIAL BEHAVIOR		
		SOCIALITY		
		TEMPERAMENT		
		TENDENCIES		
		THOUGHT PROCESSES		
		WORK		
		Psych Section Totals		
		Physical Section Totals		
		Diet Section Totals		
		GRAND TOTALS		

2. SCOLIOSIS WEEKLY SUMMARY

This table is to give you an overview of your program so that you can assess your progress and productive. Effects of dietary and exercise changes can be take months to show so this table will help monitor your progress and keep you motivated.

Reshape your spine weekly log

Metabolic type .... ○C ○M ○P
Number of Curve ○S-Shape ○C-Shape
Cobb angle .... (if applicable)

BMI at starting point ....
○ Underweight ○ Normal ○ Overweight

Start date ....

Weekly monitoring for 12 weeks	Starting point	week 1	week 2	week 3	week 4	week 5	week 6	week 7	week 8	week 9	week 10	week 11	week 12	12-week progress
Height (inch or m)														
Weight (lb or kg)														
BMI														
Angle of Trunk Rotation (ATR) using ScolioTrack		N/A		N/A		N/A		N/A		N/A		N/A		
Did you take spinal X-ray recently?	☐ yes ☐ no	N/A	N/A	N/A	N/A	N/A	N/A	N/A	N/A	N/A	N/A	N/A	N/A	
Have you mapped out your symptoms of scoliosis?	☐ yes ☐ no	N/A	N/A	N/A	☐ yes ☐ no	N/A	N/A	N/A	☐ yes ☐ no	N/A	N/A	N/A	☐ yes ☐ no	
Have you marked out your trigger points ?	☐ yes ☐ no	N/A	N/A	N/A	☐ yes ☐ no	N/A	N/A	N/A	☐ yes ☐ no	N/A	N/A	N/A	☐ yes ☐ no	

3. FOOD AND EXERCISE DIARY

To get the most out of your program I expect you to fill this table on daily basis. You will have record the foods you ate and how they made you feel as well as the types of exercises you did. This will help you determine if something is working for you and trouble shoot problems as they arise. This is why the food and exercise diary are such a vital part of this program.

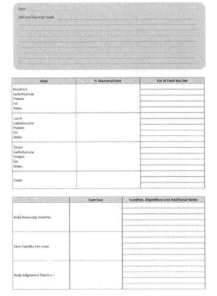

4. SCOLIOSIS MAP:

Use this diagram to mark out your scoliosis. Determine the location of the curves and how many there are in your spine. This is to be done at the beginning of the program.

Follow the steps below to map out your own scoliosis and to understand your body more closely.

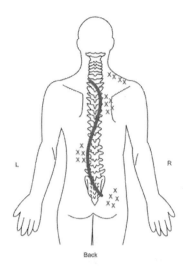

Back

How to use:

To be able to correct your scoliosis, you need to figure out your muscular symmetry and strength. You will have to first identify the muscles that feel tight and are stretched out. Following is an example of a person's back with their S-shaped scoliosis fully mapped out with muscle tightness and locations of the spinal curvature.

- First draw in your scoliosis curve — based on your latest X-rays. If you don't have an X-ray report, get another person to run his/ her finger down your spine feeling for the spinous processes (the bumps that go down your back).

- Next map out the areas of muscle tightness with an XXX. For assistance, refer to Figures 10 and 11 of my first book for the typical muscle tightness's are usually present for a S or C shaped scoliosis

5. SYMPTOMS OF SCOLIOSIS WORKSHEET:

Use this diagram to mark out any symptoms associated to your scoliosis. This is to be done once a month and can help you track any changes to these symptoms as you progress.

How to use:

In order to be able to correct your scoliosis, it is necessary to determine the muscles that are affected the most and identify the problem areas of your back where you most often experience symptoms such as pain, numbness, or pins and needles.

You can follow the below example diagram to map out your own scoliosis symptoms. It is recommended that you do this every 4 weeks so you can track any chances to your symptoms.

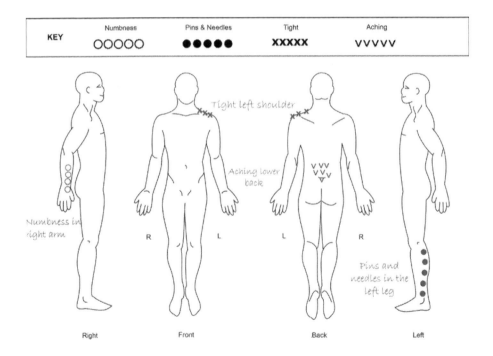

6. TRIGGER POINT WORKSHEET:

Find the trigger points associated with your scoliosis learn how to treat them by your self.

<u>How to use:</u>

Locate your trigger points so you know where to massage. Usually, you're able to feel a trigger point just by moving your fingers along a muscle until you feel an especially tight or taunt area. Keep moving along this tightness until you find the spot that's especially tender to your touch. If you move over a recently developed trigger point, the muscle twitches, but chronic trigger points just feel tight. Using the following body diagram, mark the trigger points you find.

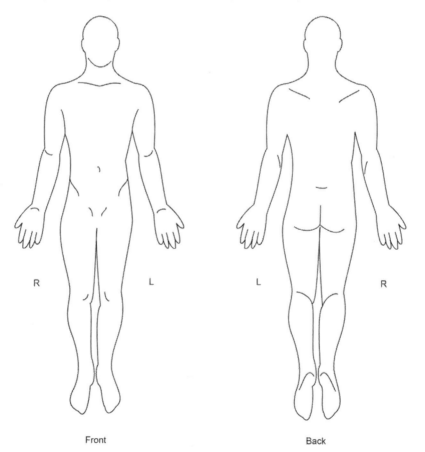

Front   Back

Additional Tips to Using this Workbook

Consistently fill your diary, which will keep you encouraged to meet goals and thereby keeps you motivated.

Here are a few tips that will help you tremendously:

1. You may come across a number of grey areas on the table. Please go ahead and read these first. These grey areas will remind you of important content that you don't want to miss.

2. If you just want to eat what you love, please make sure they are in accordance with the nutrition principles and your metabolic type (refer to shopping list on page 320-321 of *"Your Plan for Natural Scoliosis Prevention and Treatment"*).

3. Fill out the DIET RECORD SHEET on page 328 of *"Your Plan for Natural Scoliosis Prevention and Treatment"* about 2 to 3 hours after your meal. This will enable you to know how you feel after meals which will help you fine tune your diet for your metabolic type. For example, you will realize while updating the daily sheet that some foods makes you feel great after 2- 3 hours in terms of satiety, satisfaction and a pleasant effect; while some foods may make you miserable and leaves you hungry and craving. Obviously, this will give you the answer about the type and proportions of protein/carbohydrates/fat that your body needs.

4. Design your scoliosis exercise plan by following the instructions from *"Your Plan for Natural Scoliosis Prevention and Treatment"* book or *"Scoliosis Exercises for Prevention and Correction"* DVD.

5. At the last day of each week, also fill out SCOLIOSIS WEEKLY SUMMARY on page 50 for your weekly and monthly comparison.

6. If you don't know how to map out your scoliosis and its symptoms, please read chapter 12, page 196 of "**Your Plan for Natural Scoliosis Prevention and Treatment**".

7. If you don't know how to mark out the trigger points and need more guidence, please read chapter 17, page 285-289 of "**Your Plan for Natural Scoliosis Prevention and Treatment**" book.

8. Use the ScolioTrack or Scoliometer App on your iPhone, iPad or Android to measure your "Angle of Trunk Rotation" to determine the severity of your scoliosis.

9. When you are half way done with your healthy journey, i.e. 12 weeks, write down your progress on "12-week progress" column by comparing the data week by week, as well as comparing to the data of starting point.

10. On the last day of your healthy journey, write the end date on the date line. Mark the BMI range to see any change.

11. Note: Ideally at your starting point, you should have a spinal X-ray (optional), map out your symptoms of scoliosis, and mark out your trigger points. The "Yes" or "No" checkbox on the first column can make sure you do all of these without missing any of the procedures.

My Recommendations

Your health is your responsibility and you can improve the age related wear and tear changes by just modulating your methods of living and acquiring nutrition. A lot of people have relatively poor understanding and concepts about food and nutrition. Let me ask you a question:

Do you think the quality of nutrition is dependent on the amount of nutrients it contains?

If your answer is yes, I have to tell you – IT'S A WRONG ANSWER

The quality of nutrition lies in how you consume it. The methods of acquiring nutrition, cooking, portions and a lot of factors come into play that helps in determining the nutrition you are consuming is delivering high quality nutrients in your body. I am sure my recommendations below will help you in getting the most health benefits from your food.

Select the recipes from the companion cookbook, which are specific to your metabolic type and benefit to your spine health.

I suggest you to maintain a very dynamic lifestyle with ample time for physical activity every day. Moreover, make sure to choose work outs that enable you to exercise aerobically two to three times a week (e.g. brisk walking, cycling and swimming). If you have been living a sedentary lifestyle, it is high time to get your body rolling. Besides regular physical activity, other recommendations that may helps in achieving great muscular and bone health includes:

Deep tissue massage

This workbook will help in identifying your trigger points and research and clinical studies indicate that self treatment of your trigger points by deep tissue massage can stimulate natural healing processes. Let your body experience a soothing release of neurological chemicals and reset your neuromuscular system for maximum relief and an unbeatable soothing effect.

Consulting a professional:

Although the aim of this book and other content that you see online and in books is to prepare you to devise a healthy meal plan for yourself. But I still prefer to get the initial diet and exercise plan constructed by you to be evaluated by a chiropractor or spinal professional. He/she can give you professional advice to correct your spine curve and overall health.

Using screening tests to check for scoliosis in your loved-ones:

Isn't it scary to think that since scoliosis is a genetic issue, may be your family members may be suffering from it?

Isn't it much better to know or ascertain the risk before your loved ones develop complications and pain interfering with normal daily activities?

If you want to verify that your family member may suffer from scoliosis, then detect it by using HOME SCREEN on page 38-39 and ADAMS FORWARD BEND TEST on page 37 of "Your Plan for Natural Scoliosis Prevention and Treatment" book.

Pregnancy and scoliosis:

Pregnancy and pregnancy related hormonal issues can aggravate the scoliotic process in individuals. Pregnancy stop women from acquiring a lot of interventions or treatments, but I don't recommend to wait for child-birth. Yes, indeed you cannot perform regular exercises during pregnancy to correct your scoliosis lesion, but nonetheless, you may definitely want to check out my book that is especially designed for pregnant mothers and their body needs for the management of scoliosis.

Make sure to give a read to *"An Essential Guide for Scoliosis and a Healthy Pregnancy"*, which contains everything you need to know about taking care of your spine and your baby.

How to use ScolioTrack

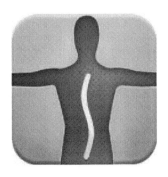

I recommend that you also use ScolioTrack, an innovative iPhone and Android application. that helps you measure a person's scoliosis or Angle of Trunk Rotation (ATR), a key measurement in screening for and planning scoliosis treatment. It also tracks a patient's height, weight, and photo record of their back; this is very beneficial for teenagers going through growth spurts or adults with degenerative scoliosis.

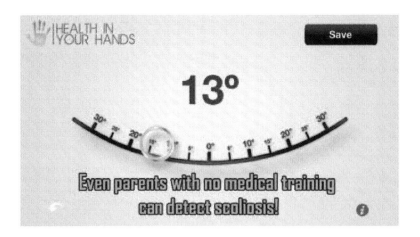

There are two steps to measure your scoliosis accurately by using ScolioTrack:

Step 1: Calibrating ScolioTrack

You can learn to use the easy and convenient ScolioTrack by following these simple steps:

1. Hold the device on the table or any flat surface with the button side of the device in the top position. Press the "**Calibrate 1**" tab.

2. Next rotate the device on the same surface and turn it to face in the opposite direction. Press "**Calibrate 2**" tab.

3. Press **Done** on the top right hand corner to end the process of calibration.

4. Press **Back** button on the bottom left corner to recalibrate, if your ScolioTrack does not read zero degree on a flat surface.

How to Measure Your Scoliosis?

In order to adequately and accurately measure your scoliosis with ScolioTrack, you will need a companion or assistant. Follow these steps:

1. The companion stand behind you while you stand in a perfectly straight position with the arms stretched in front. Slowly lean forward and bend down as far as you comfortably can.

2. Try adjusting your position for a clearer vision of the hump, protrusion or deformity in the spine.

3. The companion gently lay ScolioTrack device across the protrusion or hump and the phone needs to be centered over the spine.

4. Click on the Save button to record the Angle of Trunk Rotation or ATR which is a measure of Scoliosis (i.e. how much the spine has twisted.)

5. Now take a photo of the person back to analyze their posture on the day when the scoliosis reading is recorded. This will help in understanding the visual changes in the Scoliosis as it progresses.

6. While taking the photo, the shoulders need to be aligned with the guides marked and the patient's body in the centre.

7. It is not mandatory to update the photo, but it is definitely recommended for future reference.

8. Next enter the height and weight on the date that you have tracked the Scoliosis, using ScolioTrack. This will make tracking your progress easier.

This special feature of tracking your photos, weight and height, along with the Scoliosis degree, is a great way to monitor the Scoliosis in a growing child who's going through their growth spurt years.

9. Also, in the case of adults, it helps in tracking the changes in height and weight which are caused by degeneration or deterioration due to the worsening scoliosis every year.

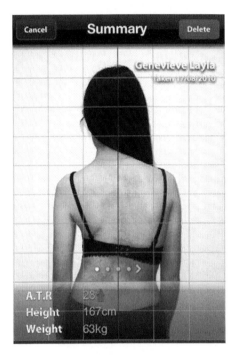 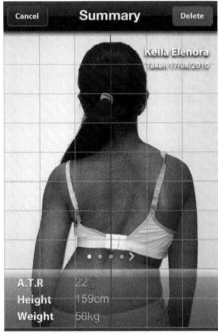

What are the benefits of using ScolioTrack?

ScolioTrack places an instrument similar to a doctor's scoliometer into your hands and is much safer than x-ray technology with high degree of accuracy. It is also simple enough for your personal use at home in between doctor's visits.

ScolioTrack saves all the information in one convenient location and provides touch of the finger retrieval for your future checkups and comparison. An easy-to-read display also displays data in graph format to easily view any changes over time.

For more information about the ScolioTrack and watch a video tutorial of how to use scoliotrack please visit: **www.scoliotrack.com**

Body Mass Index - BMI

Body composition can vary greatly from individual to individual. Two people who possess the same height and weight can have different bone structure and varying percentages of muscle and fat. Therefore, your weight alone is not the only factor in assessing your risk for weight related health issues. It has long been known that a lower BMI in adolescents is associated with greater risk of scoliosis. Adults with scoliosis can be anywhere from underweight, normal or over weight. Knowing a person's BMI can help track how the diet and exercises are progressing.

Calculating your BMI: Locate your height in the left hand column below. Then move across the row to your weight. The number at the very top the column is your BMI.

$$\text{BMI} = \frac{\text{mass}(\text{kg})}{(\text{height}(\text{m}))^2} \qquad \text{BMI} = \frac{\text{mass}(\text{lb})}{(\text{height}(\text{in}))^2} \times 703$$

BMI	19	20	21	22	23	24	25	26	27	28	29	30	31	32	33	34	35	36
Height							weight in pounds											
4'10"	91	96	100	105	110	115	119	124	129	134	138	143	148	153	158	162	167	
4'11"	94	99	104	109	114	119	124	128	133	138	143	148	153	158	163	168	173	
5'	97	102	107	112	118	123	128	133	138	143	148	153	158	163	168	174	179	
5'1"	100	106	111	116	122	127	132	137	143	148	153	158	164	169	174	180	185	
5'2"	104	109	115	120	126	131	136	142	147	153	158	164	169	175	180	186	191	
5'3"	107	113	118	124	130	135	141	146	152	158	163	169	175	180	186	191	197	
5'4"	110	116	122	128	134	140	145	151	157	163	169	174	180	186	192	197	204	
5'5"	114	120	126	132	138	144	150	156	162	168	174	180	186	192	198	204	210	
5'6"	118	124	130	136	142	148	155	161	167	173	179	186	192	198	204	210	216	
5'7"	121	127	134	140	146	153	159	166	172	178	185	191	198	204	211	217	223	
5'8"	125	131	138	144	151	158	164	171	177	184	190	197	203	210	216	223	230	
5'9"	128	135	142	149	155	162	169	176	182	189	196	203	209	216	223	230	236	
5'10"	132	139	146	153	160	167	174	181	188	195	202	209	216	222	229	236	243	
5'11"	136	143	150	157	165	172	179	186	193	200	208	215	222	229	236	243	250	
6'	140	147	154	162	169	177	184	191	199	206	213	221	226	235	242	250	258	
6'1"	144	151	159	166	174	182	189	197	204	212	219	227	235	242	250	257	265	
6'2"	148	155	163	171	179	186	194	202	210	218	225	233	241	249	256	264	272	
6'3"	152	160	168	176	184	192	200	208	216	224	232	240	248	256	264	272	279	

Healthy	Overweight	Obese

Chapter 3

Concise Scoliosis Nutrition and Exercise Program

The Top 15 Food Rules for Optimal Spine Health

In "Your Plan for Natural Scoliosis Prevention and Treatment" book I go into detail the important nutritional concepts necessary for health spinal development. Contained here is a concise guide of everything you wanted to know about protein, carbs, calories, probiotics, vitamin D, cooking oils, foods that burn fat, foods that make you fat, foods that can kill you slowly, and much more.

Before we start listing the important foods for scoliosis, let's establish the theory behind the nutritional recommendation.

The Theory Behind the Scoliosis Diet

Okay, so let's simplify nutrition a bit here... everyone out there seems confused about what is the best "diet" to be on. People seem to love to always jump from fad diet to fad diet such as low-fat diets, atkins diets, south beach diets, grapefruit diets, detox diets, vegetarian diets, and other sometimes ridiculous diets that most times are based on one person's opinion or marketing scheme (or personal agenda) rather than based on actual science.

The only "diet" that's actually based on real science is the study of paleolithic nutrition (aka paleo diet). But I hate to call it "paleo diet", because it's not like any other fad diet, since it's based on real archaeological nutritional science about what our ancestors ate before the agricultural revolution came around. The idea is simply that for the first 99.5% of our existence (ancestors back as far as 2 Million years ago, homo erectus), we only ate wild plants and animals, while for the last 0.5% of our existence (since the agricultural revolution in the last 5,000-10,000 years), humans now almost entirely eat farmed plants and animals. The biggest change this represents is the massive inclusion of grains in our current diet (and what our animals are fed) now compared to our Paleolithic ancestors.

Many people think that we don't know exactly what ancient humans ate... but this is false.

Nutritional archaeologists know pretty convincingly what ancient humans ate as they study a lot of evidence such as ancient feces remains as well as studying isotope ratios in human bone samples from all over the world through every time period in history to determine ratios of animals vs plants that ancient humans ate --which by the way, was always an omnivorous mixture of plants and animals, and a fairly high protein intake...there was no such thing as ancient paleolithic vegetarians...any Nutritional Archaelogist can confirm that they simply didn't exist. We were all omnivores that ate different ratios of plants and animals based on what part of the world, what latitude we lived, and the time of the year.

So what exactly did our Paleolithic ancestors eat for the first 99.5% of our existence, representing what we are still programmed to eat? Simple:

- Wild meat, fish, and seafood (animals that ate the right foods, unlike our current farmed meats and farmed fish)

- fruits

- vegetables

- eggs

- nuts

- seeds

Grains were only a very TINY fraction of the ancient Paleolithic diet as there was no way to process large amounts of grain back in that day into flour, so amounts of wild grain would have been small such as a few grains in an occasional soup or stew. As you can see, this is vastly different from the modern human diet that includes grain at almost every meal and in very large quantities in cereals, breads, pasta, muffins, bagels, etc.

So with that big picture explained...let's get into the details of my top 15 food rules:

Food Rule #1.

Do not eliminate carbohydrate from your diet completely as they are not bad if consumed in reasonable quantity. But processed sugars and grains are needed to be minimized. Consuming carbohydrates from vegetables can be healthy instead of processed sugar and grains. I prefer starchy vegetables that satisfy your satiety and keep you full for a longer period of time. Consuming grains like cereals, bread, pasta, bagels etc not only abuse the sugar level in blood regulation system but they also have high amount of anti nutrients which keeps the human body from engrossing minerals. Gluten also can create chronic inflammation in gut and can also damage the digestive system in certain cases.

Sweet potatoes, potatoes and other tubers can issue less digestive system inflammation problems as compared to grains. Sweet potatoes, potatoes can be tolerated better by active people and can burn off their extra carbohydrates easily.

Food Rule #2.

Always focus on good quality source of protein like wild game, seafood, wish fish, grass fed meats and free roaming organically fed eggs. Try to avoid farmed fish and farmed meat as they are mostly fed on grains and are also kept in factory environment which is unhealthy.

Food Rule #3.

Usually people are unaware of the ratio of fatty acid omega 6 to omega 3 in the food they consume. In our ancestral era of human diet the paleo followers has this ratio in the form 1:1 to 2:1 of omega 6: omega 3 fats. But in our modern diet this ratio is 20:1 to 30:1 of omega6: omega 3 fats. This is another cause of most of degenerative diseases.

To balance this ratio certain thing should be cut off from our diet like corn oils, cotton seed oils, soybean oils and should reduce the intake of grass fed meats and farmed fish as they are fed with grains. Add wild fish, grass fed dairy, grass fed meats, free range eggs and those food which contains more amount of omega 3. Walnuts, chia seeds, hemp seeds, fish oil or krill oil contains omega 3 and they are vital source of EPA and DHA. Consuming fish oil and krill oil is very beneficial as fish oil consist large quantity of EPA and DHA with high overall omega 3 volume and krill oil consist of antioxidants which is beneficial in astaxanthin and have high absorption rate as compared to fish oil.

It is important to know that omega 3 from animal sources plays healthier role in our diet as compared to plant omega 3 sources (chia, walnut and flax). It is because omega 3 in animal source already converted DHA and EPA where as plant source doesn't and our human body is not efficient in converting EPA and DHA.

Food Rule #4.

Beside processed sugar, the three worst foods which should be deducted from western diet are soy, corn and wheat with their derivatives corn syrup, soybean oil, corn oil, soy protein etc. From study it is concluded that in most of the western countries like Canada, US, Australia etc, people on average western diet plan consume approximately 67 % of corn, wheat and soy with their derivatives.

Food Rule #5.

It is important for you to know about the ingredients which cause inflammation and hidden calories in dressings and condiments. Mostly people didn't realize the fact that high calories and corn syrup high in fructose can damage the metabolism, when consumed in the form of ketchup, cocktail sauce, marinades and salad dressings etc.

For example 1 tbsp Ketchup contains 5 grams sugar and if the person eating ketchup with fries and burger then he would be consuming about 2 to 4 tbsp of ketchup which is about 10 to 20 grams of sugar just from ketchup, without counting the extra sweet drink which usually people consumed with meals.

Be a label reader and avoid HFCS! And despite deceptive advertisements out there from the corn refining industry that claim "HFCS is no worse than sugar and is natural", this is far from the truth as you can read Read Chapter 8. Essential Carbohydrates which shows why HFCS is indeed worse than plain sugar, despite them both being terrible for you.

Food Rule #6.

Some people didn't realize the fact that they are addicted to sugar which in turns damaging the body internally. Keep this in mind while consuming candies or drinking sweetened drinks that sugar can't be burned off easily. Sugar not only makes a person fat, it can cause heart disease, diabetes and can also give feed to cancer cells. It is highly recommended to avoid sugar and consume lesser amount from natural sources like fruits etc.

Food Rule #7.

Most of the canola oil companies marketed their product to be safe and healthy which also contains monounsaturated fats just like olive oil. This is not the fact, from biochemical standpoint canola oil has nothing compare to olive oil and their reaction in the body is entirely different. It is recommended to avoid canola oil completely.

Food Rule #8.

In addition to avoiding canola oil, I highly recommend avoiding soybean oil, corn oil, or cottonseed oil as much as possible too. These oils are highly inflammatory in your body, disrupt your omega-3 to omega-6 fatty acid balance in your body, and also are typically made of genetically modified crops, of which the long term health consequences are not yet fully understood by scientists.

Chapter 10. The Truth about Fats in 'Your Plan for Natural Scoliosis Prevention and Treatment' details everything you need to know about which cooking oils to fully avoid and which oils are healthy for you. You might be surprised to see why fats you falsely thought were unhealthy such as butter, lard, and coconut oil are actually the healthiest fats/oils to cook with.

Food Rule #9.

People got confused in using butter or margarine. These so called healthy margarines are not healthy at all as they are made from soybean or corn oil and are inflammatory. It is advised to add grass fed butter in your daily diet and say NO to margarines.

Food Rule #10.

Egg whites vs whole eggs? Once again, I have no idea why anyone is still debating this. Most of the general population has still not gotten the memo that egg yolks are actually the healthiest part of the egg, with over 90% of the micronutrients and antioxidants, and 100% of the fat soluble vitamins that are so important for our health. Why anybody would only eat egg whites and avoid yolks is beyond comprehension. And no, the dietary cholesterol in eggs is not bad for your heart... in fact, it increases your good HDL cholesterol. I have a full article here on why whole eggs are much healthier than egg whites, help increase your fat burning hormones, and why I personally eat 3-4 whole eggs per day and how this helps to stay in single digit body fat range.

Food Rule #11.

Remember that despite all of the bad nutrition information you hear from the government and the media, saturated fats have been falsely villified in the past, and are much healthier for you than most people realize. In fact, in recent years, scientists have become a lot more clear that saturated fats are actually important for health and hormone balance, your cell membranes, and many other vital functions in your body. You can read my article here about why saturated fats aren't so bad after all, and can even be healthy sometimes depending on source.

If you're interested in more of the actual science about why saturated fat can be healthy for you, I have an article below written by a PhD in Nutritional Biochemistry called The Truth about Saturated Fat - it's a must read if you want to understand the science about why saturated fats have been falsely villified and how to enjoy these foods that have always been part of the ancestral human diet.

Food Rule #12.

It is highly recommended to avoid artificial sweeteners as they are calorie less but very harmful for body. Many studies show that using artificial sweetener resulting in weight gain. Some new researches show that these artificial sweeteners trick the body in releasing insulin because of the cells in stomach and mouth which can sense sweetness. Keep in mind that high insulin can create fat deposition in body. Also after consuming these artificial sweeteners a person's cravings towards sugars and carbohydrates increased in few hours.

Food Rule #13.

Pay attention to your Vitamin D levels.

Vitamin D is one of the most important substances in your body. It's one of the single most important things in your body that control your hormones as well as your immune system. If you get sick often or have hormone imbalances, it's quite likely that the cause is linked to low vitamin D levels.

Unfortunately, it's estimated that almost 90% of Americans are deficient in vitamin D. Get your blood levels of vitamin D tested. Your goal should be blood levels between 50-70 ng/ml, where hormonal balance and immune function seems to be maximized. Sadly, most people typically clock in with levels in the 20's or 30's or lower, and these sub par levels can cause a lot of health problems.

Mid day sunshine is the most important source of vitamin D as your body produces vitamin D from a reaction with oils in your skin and UVB rays from the sun. Fatty fish, egg yolks, and organ meats are the best sources of dietary vitamin D, but it is hard to get enough vitamin D from diet alone, so small doses of daily mid-day sun is also important for your health (without burning).

For lots more great info on vitamin D, and it's powerful benefits to your body, you can also read a really interesting article here that shows why vitamin D can even make you the equivalent of 5 years YOUNGER!

Food Rule #14.

Probiotics rock!

Along with vitamin D levels, this is one of the single most important things you can do for your health. Your "microbiome" in your gut is made up of TRILLIONS of microbes in total and hundreds of types of these friendly probiotics. These serve so many more vitally important functions in your body than most people realize.

Probiotics are equally important to your immune system as your vitamin D levels. Probiotics are your first line of defense in keeping pathogens at bay and preventing sickness. They're extremely important for your digestion too.

Read chapter 7. Introduction to Fermented Foods to see how probiotics can improve your digestion and immunity as well as the best sources to build up your healthy colonies in your digestive system.

Food Rule #15.

Lastly, enjoy your food! And enjoy good company with food. Don't just mindlessly eat food in front of the TV. Studies show that people unknowingly eat more calories and gain more weight when they mindlessly eat in front of the TV. Instead, focus on your meal instead of a distraction...savor each bite you have. Pay attention and enjoy the subtle flavors and aroma of each bite. This makes you enjoy your food more, while eating less calories.

Designing Your Scoliosis Exercises Program

It's never been easy to switch from a sedentary life towards active life exercise program. Exercise is best for human body and a person can prevent himself from many diseases. There are 3 types of exercise available which can be effective for your spine curve.

BODY BALANCING STRETCH EXERCISE

1. Focuses on stretching to the point of feeling tension in your muscles, not to the point of pain.

2. Map your scoliosis monthly and note the areas of tightness particularly from the muscles that surround the spine.

3. If you want to increase the difficulty of the stretch and am not feeling any bad symptoms associated while doing the stretch then you can hold it longer than what is instructed. .

CORE STABILITY EXERCISES

1. Core stability exercises may be the most significant activity you can do to stabilize and support your spine.

2. Core muscle strength and stability test is pretty effective to assess your core strength and endurance over time. Keep practicing the routine three or four times each week until you can complete the test fully and comfortably.

3. Once you are able to complete the core stability test, you can move on to the beginner and advanced core stability exercises that target different areas of your core.

BODY ALIGNMENT EXERCISES

1. Body alignment exercises repeatedly strengthen the muscles around your spine which are especially beneficial in the treatment of spine-related disorders.

2. A mirror or another person should be used to observe how you perform them to make sure proper alignment of the spine.

Exercises precautions

Keep in mind:

- Listen to your body. Allow time for it to adapt to the workout.

- Do not exercise if you are not feeling well.

- Wear proper clothes to allow the skin breath and wear good, comfortable shoes for good support of the spine, hips, knees, ankles, and feet.

- Don't forget to warm up prior to stretching.

- If the muscle group being stretched isn't 100% healthy, avoid stretching this area altogether. Work on recovery and rehabilitation as the first priority.

- If, during exercise, you experience any pain or discomfort that does not go away after 15 minutes, stop the exercise and call your doctor.

- Never over-train.

- Cooling down and stretching after exercise or physical activity is just as important as a warm up.

- Avoid exercising strenuously during heat waves and humid weather.

- Drink plenty of fluids before, during, and after your exercise regimen.

Plan for your workout

A well-balanced exercise program can improve your general health, develop your endurance, and enhance your emotional well-being. A workout plan should be tailored to your needs, goals, and suit your lifestyle pattern.

Firstly, you should assess your situation:

- How much time do you devote to exercise every day?

- If you are a working person and worry about your physical power, I can tell you, scientists revealed that people who exercise on work days are more productive, happier, and suffer less stress than on non-workout days.

- What physical activities do you enjoy?

  Finding activities you enjoy and find to be fun are the best.

- Where will you workout?

  Find the most convenient place for your exercises and your plan execution.

- What equipments do you need for workout?

  Sometimes what you have is pretty average, just a ball, a table, but what you do with it may become an advantage.

Make a weekly workout plan for obtaining a monthly goal and tailor your activities along with your mood, feelings and availability.

The following is an example of a weekly workout plan. Read chapter 14-18 in "Your Plan for Natural Scoliosis Prevention and Treatment" to help you understand your body and schedule your plan.

Remember: 10 minutes warm-up and cool-down before and after the exercise.

Physical activities include which you can also include in your scoliosis exercise plan should focus on low intesity. These exercises include but not limited to:

- Bicycling

- Stationary

- Water activities, such as swimming

- Brisk walking

- Stair climbing

- Yoga or pilates

The only bad workout is the one that didn't happen.

Setting Weekly Goals

At the beginning of each week, your journal has a section where you can set some nutritional and exercise goals. These goals should be specific and measureable. For example rather than aim to "cut back on sweets," set a goal to "limit to one sweet per day" or "switch from sodas to mineral water." Instead of "exercise more," write "complete level 1 plank holding for 60 sec" or "add 2 new body balancing stretches."

Make sure your goals are sensible! If your use to eating a bowl of rice or bread for dinner every night, don't suddenly cut out all bread or rice; instead try setting a goal of half portion which would be a more practical goal. If you typically exercise twice a week, aim for three sessions rather than six.

You needn't push yourself to new heights every week. Sometimes, its best to stick with the same goal for several weeks, or even months, until the practice becomes a habit and you're ready to reach for the next level. At other times, however, you might be in the mood to really test yourself. Maybe this is the week you're determined to following your metabolic type for all your breakfasts. Also consider your personality. Some people succeed when their goals are moderately challenging whereas others thrive when they shoot for the stars.

Days of the week	Workout	Intensity	Duration	Monthly goal
Monday	Bicycling	light	15-30 min	40 min
Tuesday	4 Body Balancing Stretches, 4 Core Stability Exercises and 3 Body Alignment Exercises	Follow the DVD and book instructions to exercise.		
Wednesday	Swimming	light	15-30 min	40 min
Thursday	4 Body Balancing Stretches, 4 Core Stability Exercises and 3 Body Alignment Exercises	Follow the DVD and book instructions to exercise.		
Friday	Yoga	moderate	15-30 min	40 min
Saturday	Rest day	N/A		
Sunday	4 Body Balancing Stretches, 4 Core Stability Exercises and 3 Body Alignment Exercises	Follow the DVD and book instructions to exercise.		

Example of Weekly Exercise Schedule

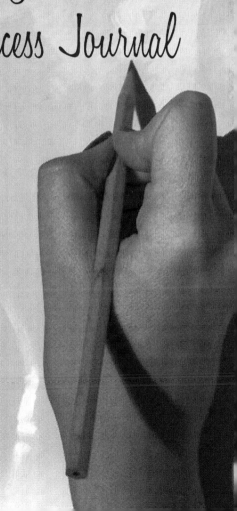

PART 2 Day-by-Day
Scoliosis Success Journal

Reshape your spine weekly log

Start date _____

Metabolic type ○ Carbo Type   ○ Mixed Type   ○ Protien Type
Number of Curve _____   ○ S-Shape   ○ C-Shape
Cobb angle _____ (If applicable)

BMI at starting point _____
○ Underweight   ○ Normal   ○ Overweight

Weekly monitoring for 12 weeks	Starting point	week 1	week 2	week 3	week 4	week 5	week 6	week 7	week 8	week 9	week 10	week 11	week 12	12-week progress
Height (inch or m)														
Weight (lb or kg)														
BMI														
Angle of Trunk Rotation (ATR) using ScolioTrack		N/A	N/A		N/A	N/A	N/A		N/A	N/A	N/A		N/A	
Did you take spinal X-ray recently?	☐ yes ☐ no	N/A	N/A	N/A	☐ yes ☐ no	N/A	N/A	N/A	☐ yes ☐ no	N/A	N/A	N/A	☐ yes ☐ no	
Have you mapped out your symptoms of scoliosis?	☐ yes ☐ no	N/A	N/A	N/A	☐ yes ☐ no	N/A	N/A	N/A	☐ yes ☐ no	N/A	N/A	N/A	☐ yes ☐ no	
Have you marked out your trigger points ?	☐ yes ☐ no	N/A	N/A	N/A	☐ yes ☐ no	N/A	N/A	N/A	☐ yes ☐ no	N/A	N/A	N/A	☐ yes ☐ no	

Week 1: Scoliosis Map

Refer to Chapter 12 in *"Your Plan for Natural Scoliosis Prevention and Treatment"* to learn how to map your scoliosis. By familarising your self with your scoliosis and where it bends it can help you design the right exercises for you.

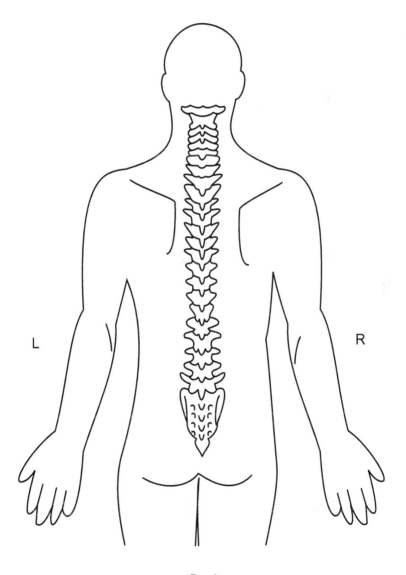

L   R

Back

Week 1: Scoliosis Symptoms Review

In order to be able to correct your scoliosis, it is necessary to determine which muscles are affected, and identify the areas of your back where you most often experience symptoms such as pain, numbness or pins and needles. in *"**Your Plan for Natural Scoliosis Prevention and Treatment**"* learn how to map the symptoms associated with your scoliosis. You will do this review every 4 weeks to monitor your progress and note any changes in your symptoms while you correct your scoliosis.

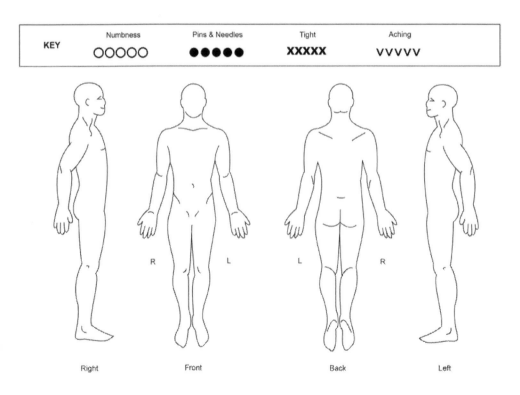

Week 1: Trigger Point Mapping

Refer to Chapter 17. Living with Scoliosis in *"**Your Plan for Natural Scoliosis Prevention and Treatment**"* to learn how to map your Trigger Points. Work on these trigger points on 2-3 times a week to see improvements to muscle imbalances and pain. Fill out the trigger point diagram every 4 weeks to monitor your progress.

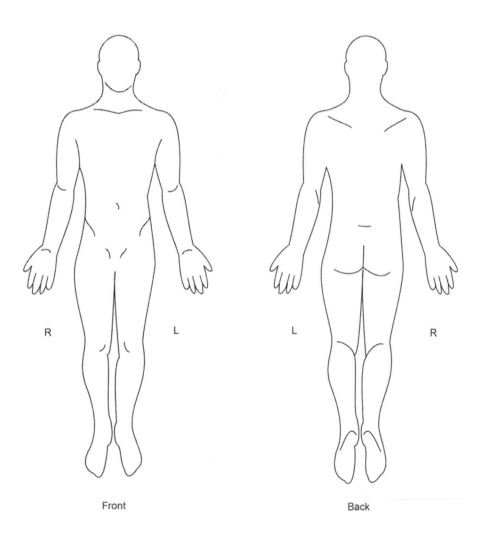

Front   Back

DIET AND EXERCISE JOURNAL   WEEK 1 / DAY 1

Date : _____

Diet and Exercise Goals : _____

_____

_____

_____

_____

Meal	List of Food You Ate	Additional Notes
Breakfast		
Lunch		
Dinner		
Snack		

	Exercises	Duration, Repetitions and Additional Notes
Body Balancing Streches		
Core Stability Exercises		
Body Allignment Exercises		

> When someone tells me "no," it doesn't mean I can't do it, it simply means I can't do it with them.
> - Karen E. Quinones Miller

Diet Record Sheet	☐Breakfast ☐Lunch ☐Dinner	
Reactions after a meal	**Good**	**Bad**
APPETITE FULLNESS / SATISFACTION SWEET CRAVINGS	Following the meal . . . ☐ Feel full, satisfied ☐ Do NOT have sweet cravings ☐ Do NOT desire more food ☐ Do NOT get hungry soon after ☐ Do NOT need to snack before next meal	Following the meal . . . ☐ Feel physically full, but still hungry ☐ Don't feel satisfied; feel like something was missing from meal ☐ Have desire for sweets ☐ Feel hungry again soon after meal ☐ Need to snack between meals
ENERGY LEVELS	Normal energy response to meal: ☐ Energy is restored after eating ☐ Have good, lasting, "normal" sense of energy and well-being	Poor energy response to meal: ☐ Too much or too little energy ☐ Become hyper, jittery, shaky, nervous, or speedy ☐ Feel hyper, but exhausted "underneath" ☐ Energy drop, fatigue, exhaustion, sleepiness, drowsiness, lethargy, or listlessness
MENTAL EMOTIONAL WELL-BEING	Normal qualities: ☐ Improved well-being ☐ Sense of feeling refueled and restored ☐ Upliftment in emotions ☐ Improved clarity and acuity of mind ☐ Normalization of thought processes	Abnormal qualities: ☐ Mentally slow, sluggish, spacey ☐ Inability to think quickly or clearly ☐ Hyper, overly rapid thoughts ☐ Inability to focus/hold attention ☐ Hypo traits: Apathy, depression, sadness ☐ Hyper traits: Anxious, obsessive, fearful, angry, short tempered, or irritable, etc.

DIET AND EXERCISE JOURNAL WEEK 1 / DAY 2

Date : _____

Diet and Exercise Goals : _____

_____

_____

_____

_____

Meal	List of Food You Ate	Additional Notes
Breakfast		
Lunch		
Dinner		
Snack		

	Exercises	Duration, Repetitions and Additional Notes
Body Balancing Streches		
Core Stability Exercises		
Body Allignment Exercises		

Believe that life is worth living and your belief will help create the fact. - William James

Diet Record Sheet	☐Breakfast ☐Lunch ☐Dinner	
Reactions after a meal	Good	Bad
APPETITE FULLNESS / SATISFACTION SWEET CRAVINGS	Following the meal . . . ☐ Feel full, satisfied ☐ Do NOT have sweet cravings ☐ Do NOT desire more food ☐ Do NOT get hungry soon after ☐ Do NOT need to snack before next meal	Following the meal . . . ☐ Feel physically full, but still hungry ☐ Don't feel satisfied; feel like something was missing from meal ☐ Have desire for sweets ☐ Feel hungry again soon after meal ☐ Need to snack between meals
ENERGY LEVELS	Normal energy response to meal: ☐ Energy is restored after eating ☐ Have good, lasting, "normal" sense of energy and well-being	Poor energy response to meal: ☐ Too much or too little energy ☐ Become hyper, jittery, shaky, nervous, or speedy ☐ Feel hyper, but exhausted "underneath" ☐ Energy drop, fatigue, exhaustion, sleepiness, drowsiness, lethargy, or listlessness
MENTAL EMOTIONAL WELL-BEING	Normal qualities: ☐ Improved well-being ☐ Sense of feeling refueled and restored ☐ Upliftment in emotions ☐ Improved clarity and acuity of mind ☐ Normalization of thought processes	Abnormal qualities: ☐ Mentally slow, sluggish, spacey ☐ Inability to think quickly or clearly ☐ Hyper, overly rapid thoughts ☐ Inability to focus/hold attention ☐ Hypo traits: Apathy, depression, sadness ☐ Hyper traits: Anxious, obsessive, fearful, angry, short tempered, or irritable, etc.

DIET AND EXERCISE JOURNAL   WEEK 1 / DAY 3

Date : _____

Diet and Exercise Goals : _____

_____

_____

_____

_____

Meal	List of Food You Ate	Additional Notes
Breakfast		
Lunch		
Dinner		
Snack		

	Exercises	Duration, Repetitions and Additional Notes
Body Balancing Streches		
Core Stability Exercises		
Body Allignment Exercises		

Your present circumstances don't determine where you can go; they merely determine where you start. - Nido Qubein

Diet Record Sheet	☐Breakfast ☐Lunch ☐Dinner	
Reactions after a meal	Good	Bad
APPETITE FULLNESS / SATISFACTION SWEET CRAVINGS	Following the meal . . . ☐ Feel full, satisfied ☐ Do NOT have sweet cravings ☐ Do NOT desire more food ☐ Do NOT get hungry soon after ☐ Do NOT need to snack before next meal	Following the meal . . . ☐ Feel physically full, but still hungry ☐ Don't feel satisfied; feel like something was missing from meal ☐ Have desire for sweets ☐ Feel hungry again soon after meal ☐ Need to snack between meals
ENERGY LEVELS	Normal energy response to meal: ☐ Energy is restored after eating ☐ Have good, lasting, "normal" sense of energy and well-being	Poor energy response to meal: ☐ Too much or too little energy ☐ Become hyper, jittery, shaky, nervous, or speedy ☐ Feel hyper, but exhausted "underneath" ☐ Energy drop, fatigue, exhaustion, sleepiness, drowsiness, lethargy, or listlessness
MENTAL EMOTIONAL WELL-BEING	Normal qualities: ☐ Improved well-being ☐ Sense of feeling refueled and restored ☐ Upliftment in emotions ☐ Improved clarity and acuity of mind ☐ Normalization of thought processes	Abnormal qualities: ☐ Mentally slow, sluggish, spacey ☐ Inability to think quickly or clearly ☐ Hyper, overly rapid thoughts ☐ Inability to focus/hold attention ☐ Hypo traits: Apathy, depression, sadness ☐ Hyper traits: Anxious, obsessive, fearful, angry, short tempered, or irritable, etc.

DIET AND EXERCISE JOURNAL   WEEK 1 / DAY 4

Date : _____

Diet and Exercise Goals : _____

_____

_____

_____

_____

Meal	List of Food You Ate	Additional Notes
Breakfast		
Lunch		
Dinner		
Snack		

	Exercises	Duration, Repetitions and Additional Notes
Body Balancing Streches		
Core Stability Exercises		
Body Allignment Exercises		

First say to yourself what you would be; and then do what you have to do. - Epictetus

Diet Record Sheet		☐Breakfast ☐Lunch ☐Dinner
Reactions after a meal	**Good**	**Bad**
APPETITE FULLNESS / SATISFACTION SWEET CRAVINGS	Following the meal . . . ☐ Feel full, satisfied ☐ Do NOT have sweet cravings ☐ Do NOT desire more food ☐ Do NOT get hungry soon after ☐ Do NOT need to snack before next meal	Following the meal . . . ☐ Feel physically full, but still hungry ☐ Don't feel satisfied; feel like something was missing from meal ☐ Have desire for sweets ☐ Feel hungry again soon after meal ☐ Need to snack between meals
ENERGY LEVELS	Normal energy response to meal: ☐ Energy is restored after eating ☐ Have good, lasting, "normal" sense of energy and well-being	Poor energy response to meal: ☐ Too much or too little energy ☐ Become hyper, jittery, shaky, nervous, or speedy ☐ Feel hyper, but exhausted "underneath" ☐ Energy drop, fatigue, exhaustion, sleepiness, drowsiness, lethargy, or listlessness
MENTAL EMOTIONAL WELL-BEING	Normal qualities: ☐ Improved well-being ☐ Sense of feeling refueled and restored ☐ Upliftment in emotions ☐ Improved clarity and acuity of mind ☐ Normalization of thought processes	Abnormal qualities: ☐ Mentally slow, sluggish, spacey ☐ Inability to think quickly or clearly ☐ Hyper, overly rapid thoughts ☐ Inability to focus/hold attention ☐ Hypo traits: Apathy, depression, sadness ☐ Hyper traits: Anxious, obsessive, fearful, angry, short tempered, or irritable, etc.

DIET AND EXERCISE JOURNAL   WEEK 1 / DAY 5

Date : _____

Diet and Exercise Goals : _____

_____

_____

_____

_____

Meal	List of Food You Ate	Additional Notes
Breakfast		
Lunch		
Dinner		
Snack		

	Exercises	Duration, Repetitions and Additional Notes
Body Balancing Streches		
Core Stability Exercises		
Body Allignment Exercises		

That which doesn't kill us makes us stronger. - Friedrich Nietzsche

Diet Record Sheet	☐Breakfast ☐Lunch ☐Dinner	
Reactions after a meal	Good	Bad
APPETITE FULLNESS / SATISFACTION SWEET CRAVINGS	Following the meal . . . ☐ Feel full, satisfied ☐ Do NOT have sweet cravings ☐ Do NOT desire more food ☐ Do NOT get hungry soon after ☐ Do NOT need to snack before next meal	Following the meal . . . ☐ Feel physically full, but still hungry ☐ Don't feel satisfied; feel like something was missing from meal ☐ Have desire for sweets ☐ Feel hungry again soon after meal ☐ Need to snack between meals
ENERGY LEVELS	Normal energy response to meal: ☐ Energy is restored after eating ☐ Have good, lasting, "normal" sense of energy and well-being	Poor energy response to meal: ☐ Too much or too little energy ☐ Become hyper, jittery, shaky, nervous, or speedy ☐ Feel hyper, but exhausted "underneath" ☐ Energy drop, fatigue, exhaustion, sleepiness, drowsiness, lethargy, or listlessness
MENTAL EMOTIONAL WELL-BEING	Normal qualities: ☐ Improved well-being ☐ Sense of feeling refueled and restored ☐ Upliftment in emotions ☐ Improved clarity and acuity of mind ☐ Normalization of thought processes	Abnormal qualities: ☐ Mentally slow, sluggish, spacey ☐ Inability to think quickly or clearly ☐ Hyper, overly rapid thoughts ☐ Inability to focus/hold attention ☐ Hypo traits: Apathy, depression, sadness ☐ Hyper traits: Anxious, obsessive, fearful, angry, short tempered, or irritable, etc.

DIET AND EXERCISE JOURNAL   WEEK 1 / DAY 6

Date : _____

Diet and Exercise Goals : _____

_____

_____

_____

_____

Meal	List of Food You Ate	Additional Notes
Breakfast		
Lunch		
Dinner		
Snack		

	Exercises	Duration, Repetitions and Additional Notes
Body Balancing Streches		
Core Stability Exercises		
Body Allignment Exercises		

A life spent making mistakes is not only more honorable,
but more useful than a life spent doing nothing. - George Bernard Shaw

Diet Record Sheet	☐Breakfast ☐Lunch ☐Dinner	
Reactions after a meal	Good	Bad
APPETITE FULLNESS / SATISFACTION SWEET CRAVINGS	Following the meal . . . ☐ Feel full, satisfied ☐ Do NOT have sweet cravings ☐ Do NOT desire more food ☐ Do NOT get hungry soon after ☐ Do NOT need to snack before next meal	Following the meal . . . ☐ Feel physically full, but still hungry ☐ Don't feel satisfied; feel like something was missing from meal ☐ Have desire for sweets ☐ Feel hungry again soon after meal ☐ Need to snack between meals
ENERGY LEVELS	Normal energy response to meal: ☐ Energy is restored after eating ☐ Have good, lasting, "normal" sense of energy and well-being	Poor energy response to meal: ☐ Too much or too little energy ☐ Become hyper, jittery, shaky, nervous, or speedy ☐ Feel hyper, but exhausted "underneath" ☐ Energy drop, fatigue, exhaustion, sleepiness, drowsiness, lethargy, or listlessness
MENTAL EMOTIONAL WELL-BEING	Normal qualities: ☐ Improved well-being ☐ Sense of feeling refueled and restored ☐ Upliftment in emotions ☐ Improved clarity and acuity of mind ☐ Normalization of thought processes	Abnormal qualities: ☐ Mentally slow, sluggish, spacey ☐ Inability to think quickly or clearly ☐ Hyper, overly rapid thoughts ☐ Inability to focus/hold attention ☐ Hypo traits: Apathy, depression, sadness ☐ Hyper traits: Anxious, obsessive, fearful, angry, short tempered, or irritable, etc.

DIET AND EXERCISE JOURNAL   WEEK 1 / DAY 7

Date : _____

Diet and Exercise Goals : _____

_____

_____

_____

_____

Meal	List of Food You Ate	Additional Notes
Breakfast		
Lunch		
Dinner		
Snack		

	Exercises	Duration, Repetitions and Additional Notes
Body Balancing Streches		
Core Stability Exercises		
Body Allignment Exercises		

Life isn't about finding yourself. Life is about creating yourself. - George Bernard Shaw

Diet Record Sheet	☐Breakfast ☐Lunch ☐Dinner	
Reactions after a meal	Good	Bad
APPETITE FULLNESS / SATISFACTION SWEET CRAVINGS	Following the meal . . . ☐ Feel full, satisfied ☐ Do NOT have sweet cravings ☐ Do NOT desire more food ☐ Do NOT get hungry soon after ☐ Do NOT need to snack before next meal	Following the meal . . . ☐ Feel physically full, but still hungry ☐ Don't feel satisfied; feel like something was missing from meal ☐ Have desire for sweets ☐ Feel hungry again soon after meal ☐ Need to snack between meals
ENERGY LEVELS	Normal energy response to meal: ☐ Energy is restored after eating ☐ Have good, lasting, "normal" sense of energy and well-being	Poor energy response to meal: ☐ Too much or too little energy ☐ Become hyper, jittery, shaky, nervous, or speedy ☐ Feel hyper, but exhausted "underneath" ☐ Energy drop, fatigue, exhaustion, sleepiness, drowsiness, lethargy, or listlessness
MENTAL EMOTIONAL WELL-BEING	Normal qualities: ☐ Improved well-being ☐ Sense of feeling refueled and restored ☐ Upliftment in emotions ☐ Improved clarity and acuity of mind ☐ Normalization of thought processes	Abnormal qualities: ☐ Mentally slow, sluggish, spacey ☐ Inability to think quickly or clearly ☐ Hyper, overly rapid thoughts ☐ Inability to focus/hold attention ☐ Hypo traits: Apathy, depression, sadness ☐ Hyper traits: Anxious, obsessive, fearful, angry, short tempered, or irritable, etc.

DIET AND EXERCISE JOURNAL   WEEK 2 / DAY 8

Date : _____

Diet and Exercise Goals : _____

_____

_____

_____

_____

Meal	List of Food You Ate	Additional Notes
Breakfast		
Lunch		
Dinner		
Snack		

	Exercises	Duration, Repetitions and Additional Notes
Body Balancing Streches		
Core Stability Exercises		
Body Allignment Exercises		

A journey of a thousand miles begins with a single step. - Lao Tzu

Diet Record Sheet	☐Breakfast ☐Lunch ☐Dinner	
Reactions after a meal	**Good**	**Bad**
APPETITE FULLNESS / SATISFACTION SWEET CRAVINGS	Following the meal . . . ☐ Feel full, satisfied ☐ Do NOT have sweet cravings ☐ Do NOT desire more food ☐ Do NOT get hungry soon after ☐ Do NOT need to snack before next meal	Following the meal . . . ☐ Feel physically full, but still hungry ☐ Don't feel satisfied; feel like something was missing from meal ☐ Have desire for sweets ☐ Feel hungry again soon after meal ☐ Need to snack between meals
ENERGY LEVELS	Normal energy response to meal: ☐ Energy is restored after eating ☐ Have good, lasting, "normal" sense of energy and well-being	Poor energy response to meal: ☐ Too much or too little energy ☐ Become hyper, jittery, shaky, nervous, or speedy ☐ Feel hyper, but exhausted "underneath" ☐ Energy drop, fatigue, exhaustion, sleepiness, drowsiness, lethargy, or listlessness
MENTAL EMOTIONAL WELL-BEING	Normal qualities: ☐ Improved well-being ☐ Sense of feeling refueled and restored ☐ Upliftment in emotions ☐ Improved clarity and acuity of mind ☐ Normalization of thought processes	Abnormal qualities: ☐ Mentally slow, sluggish, spacey ☐ Inability to think quickly or clearly ☐ Hyper, overly rapid thoughts ☐ Inability to focus/hold attention ☐ Hypo traits: Apathy, depression, sadness ☐ Hyper traits: Anxious, obsessive, fearful, angry, short tempered, or irritable, etc.

DIET AND EXERCISE JOURNAL   WEEK 2 / DAY 9

Date : _____

Diet and Exercise Goals : _____

_____

_____

_____

_____

Meal	List of Food You Ate	Additional Notes
Breakfast		
Lunch		
Dinner		
Snack		

	Exercises	Duration, Repetitions and Additional Notes
Body Balancing Streches		
Core Stability Exercises		
Body Allignment Exercises		

You only live once, but if you do it right, once is enough. - Mae West

Diet Record Sheet	☐Breakfast ☐Lunch ☐Dinner	
Reactions after a meal	Good	Bad
APPETITE FULLNESS / SATISFACTION SWEET CRAVINGS	Following the meal . . . ☐ Feel full, satisfied ☐ Do NOT have sweet cravings ☐ Do NOT desire more food ☐ Do NOT get hungry soon after ☐ Do NOT need to snack before next meal	Following the meal . . . ☐ Feel physically full, but still hungry ☐ Don't feel satisfied; feel like something was missing from meal ☐ Have desire for sweets ☐ Feel hungry again soon after meal ☐ Need to snack between meals
ENERGY LEVELS	Normal energy response to meal: ☐ Energy is restored after eating ☐ Have good, lasting, "normal" sense of energy and well-being	Poor energy response to meal: ☐ Too much or too little energy ☐ Become hyper, jittery, shaky, nervous, or speedy ☐ Feel hyper, but exhausted "underneath" ☐ Energy drop, fatigue, exhaustion, sleepiness, drowsiness, lethargy, or listlessness
MENTAL EMOTIONAL WELL-BEING	Normal qualities: ☐ Improved well-being ☐ Sense of feeling refueled and restored ☐ Upliftment in emotions ☐ Improved clarity and acuity of mind ☐ Normalization of thought processes	Abnormal qualities: ☐ Mentally slow, sluggish, spacey ☐ Inability to think quickly or clearly ☐ Hyper, overly rapid thoughts ☐ Inability to focus/hold attention ☐ Hypo traits: Apathy, depression, sadness ☐ Hyper traits: Anxious, obsessive, fearful, angry, short tempered, or irritable, etc.

DIET AND EXERCISE JOURNAL   WEEK 2 / DAY 10

Date : _____

Diet and Exercise Goals : _____

_____

_____

_____

_____

Meal	List of Food You Ate	Additional Notes
Breakfast		
Lunch		
Dinner		
Snack		

	Exercises	Duration, Repetitions and Additional Notes
Body Balancing Streches		
Core Stability Exercises		
Body Allignment Exercises		

There are only two ways to live your life. One is as though nothing is a miracle.
The other is as though everything is a miracle. - Albert Einstein

Diet Record Sheet	☐Breakfast ☐Lunch ☐Dinner	
Reactions after a meal	Good	Bad
APPETITE FULLNESS / SATISFACTION SWEET CRAVINGS	Following the meal . . . ☐ Feel full, satisfied ☐ Do NOT have sweet cravings ☐ Do NOT desire more food ☐ Do NOT get hungry soon after ☐ Do NOT need to snack before next meal	Following the meal . . . ☐ Feel physically full, but still hungry ☐ Don't feel satisfied; feel like something was missing from meal ☐ Have desire for sweets ☐ Feel hungry again soon after meal ☐ Need to snack between meals
ENERGY LEVELS	Normal energy response to meal: ☐ Energy is restored after eating ☐ Have good, lasting, "normal" sense of energy and well-being	Poor energy response to meal: ☐ Too much or too little energy ☐ Become hyper, jittery, shaky, nervous, or speedy ☐ Feel hyper, but exhausted "underneath" ☐ Energy drop, fatigue, exhaustion, sleepiness, drowsiness, lethargy, or listlessness
MENTAL EMOTIONAL WELL-BEING	Normal qualities: ☐ Improved well-being ☐ Sense of feeling refueled and restored ☐ Upliftment in emotions ☐ Improved clarity and acuity of mind ☐ Normalization of thought processes	Abnormal qualities: ☐ Mentally slow, sluggish, spacey ☐ Inability to think quickly or clearly ☐ Hyper, overly rapid thoughts ☐ Inability to focus/hold attention ☐ Hypo traits: Apathy, depression, sadness ☐ Hyper traits: Anxious, obsessive, fearful, angry, short tempered, or irritable, etc.

DIET AND EXERCISE JOURNAL   WEEK 2 / DAY 11

Date : _____

Diet and Exercise Goals : _____

_____

_____

_____

_____

Meal	List of Food You Ate	Additional Notes
Breakfast		
Lunch		
Dinner		
Snack		

	Exercises	Duration, Repetitions and Additional Notes
Body Balancing Streches		
Core Stability Exercises		
Body Allignment Exercises		

The way to get started is to quit talking and begin doing. - Walt Disney Company

Diet Record Sheet	☐Breakfast ☐Lunch ☐Dinner	
Reactions after a meal	Good	Bad
APPETITE FULLNESS / SATISFACTION SWEET CRAVINGS	Following the meal . . . ☐ Feel full, satisfied ☐ Do NOT have sweet cravings ☐ Do NOT desire more food ☐ Do NOT get hungry soon after ☐ Do NOT need to snack before next meal	Following the meal . . . ☐ Feel physically full, but still hungry ☐ Don't feel satisfied; feel like something was missing from meal ☐ Have desire for sweets ☐ Feel hungry again soon after meal ☐ Need to snack between meals
ENERGY LEVELS	Normal energy response to meal: ☐ Energy is restored after eating ☐ Have good, lasting, "normal" sense of energy and well-being	Poor energy response to meal: ☐ Too much or too little energy ☐ Become hyper, jittery, shaky, nervous, or speedy ☐ Feel hyper, but exhausted "underneath" ☐ Energy drop, fatigue, exhaustion, sleepiness, drowsiness, lethargy, or listlessness
MENTAL EMOTIONAL WELL-BEING	Normal qualities: ☐ Improved well-being ☐ Sense of feeling refueled and restored ☐ Upliftment in emotions ☐ Improved clarity and acuity of mind ☐ Normalization of thought processes	Abnormal qualities: ☐ Mentally slow, sluggish, spacey ☐ Inability to think quickly or clearly ☐ Hyper, overly rapid thoughts ☐ Inability to focus/hold attention ☐ Hypo traits: Apathy, depression, sadness ☐ Hyper traits: Anxious, obsessive, fearful, angry, short tempered, or irritable, etc.

DIET AND EXERCISE JOURNAL   WEEK 2 / DAY 12

Date : _____

Diet and Exercise Goals : _____

_____

_____

_____

_____

Meal	List of Food You Ate	Additional Notes
Breakfast		
Lunch		
Dinner		
Snack		

	Exercises	Duration, Repetitions and Additional Notes
Body Balancing Streches		
Core Stability Exercises		
Body Allignment Exercises		

You may be disappointed if you fail, but you are doomed if you don't try. - Beverly Sills

Diet Record Sheet	☐Breakfast ☐Lunch ☐Dinner	
Reactions after a meal	**Good**	**Bad**
APPETITE FULLNESS / SATISFACTION SWEET CRAVINGS	Following the meal . . . ☐ Feel full, satisfied ☐ Do NOT have sweet cravings ☐ Do NOT desire more food ☐ Do NOT get hungry soon after ☐ Do NOT need to snack before next meal	Following the meal . . . ☐ Feel physically full, but still hungry ☐ Don't feel satisfied; feel like something was missing from meal ☐ Have desire for sweets ☐ Feel hungry again soon after meal ☐ Need to snack between meals
ENERGY LEVELS	Normal energy response to meal: ☐ Energy is restored after eating ☐ Have good, lasting, "normal" sense of energy and well-being	Poor energy response to meal: ☐ Too much or too little energy ☐ Become hyper, jittery, shaky, nervous, or speedy ☐ Feel hyper, but exhausted "underneath" ☐ Energy drop, fatigue, exhaustion, sleepiness, drowsiness, lethargy, or listlessness
MENTAL EMOTIONAL WELL-BEING	Normal qualities: ☐ Improved well-being ☐ Sense of feeling refueled and restored ☐ Upliftment in emotions ☐ Improved clarity and acuity of mind ☐ Normalization of thought processes	Abnormal qualities: ☐ Mentally slow, sluggish, spacey ☐ Inability to think quickly or clearly ☐ Hyper, overly rapid thoughts ☐ Inability to focus/hold attention ☐ Hypo traits: Apathy, depression, sadness ☐ Hyper traits: Anxious, obsessive, fearful, angry, short tempered, or irritable, etc.

DIET AND EXERCISE JOURNAL   WEEK 2 / DAY 13

Date : _____

Diet and Exercise Goals : _____

_____

_____

_____

_____

Meal	List of Food You Ate	Additional Notes
Breakfast		
Lunch		
Dinner		
Snack		

	Exercises	Duration, Repetitions and Additional Notes
Body Balancing Streches		
Core Stability Exercises		
Body Allignment Exercises		

Knowing yourself is the beginning of all wisdom. - Aristotle

Diet Record Sheet	☐Breakfast ☐Lunch ☐Dinner	
Reactions after a meal	Good	Bad
APPETITE FULLNESS / SATISFACTION SWEET CRAVINGS	Following the meal . . . ☐ Feel full, satisfied ☐ Do NOT have sweet cravings ☐ Do NOT desire more food ☐ Do NOT get hungry soon after ☐ Do NOT need to snack before next meal	Following the meal . . . ☐ Feel physically full, but still hungry ☐ Don't feel satisfied; feel like something was missing from meal ☐ Have desire for sweets ☐ Feel hungry again soon after meal ☐ Need to snack between meals
ENERGY LEVELS	Normal energy response to meal: ☐ Energy is restored after eating ☐ Have good, lasting, "normal" sense of energy and well-being	Poor energy response to meal: ☐ Too much or too little energy ☐ Become hyper, jittery, shaky, nervous, or speedy ☐ Feel hyper, but exhausted "underneath" ☐ Energy drop, fatigue, exhaustion, sleepiness, drowsiness, lethargy, or listlessness
MENTAL EMOTIONAL WELL-BEING	Normal qualities: ☐ Improved well-being ☐ Sense of feeling refueled and restored ☐ Upliftment in emotions ☐ Improved clarity and acuity of mind ☐ Normalization of thought processes	Abnormal qualities: ☐ Mentally slow, sluggish, spacey ☐ Inability to think quickly or clearly ☐ Hyper, overly rapid thoughts ☐ Inability to focus/hold attention ☐ Hypo traits: Apathy, depression, sadness ☐ Hyper traits: Anxious, obsessive, fearful, angry, short tempered, or irritable, etc.

DIET AND EXERCISE JOURNAL   WEEK 2 / DAY 14

Date : _____

Diet and Exercise Goals : _____

_____

_____

_____

_____

Meal	List of Food You Ate	Additional Notes
Breakfast		
Lunch		
Dinner		
Snack		

	Exercises	Duration, Repetitions and Additional Notes
Body Balancing Streches		
Core Stability Exercises		
Body Allignment Exercises		

It is never too late to be what you might have been. - George Eliot

Diet Record Sheet	☐Breakfast ☐Lunch ☐Dinner	
Reactions after a meal	**Good**	**Bad**
APPETITE FULLNESS / SATISFACTION SWEET CRAVINGS	Following the meal . . . ☐ Feel full, satisfied ☐ Do NOT have sweet cravings ☐ Do NOT desire more food ☐ Do NOT get hungry soon after ☐ Do NOT need to snack before next meal	Following the meal . . . ☐ Feel physically full, but still hungry ☐ Don't feel satisfied; feel like something was missing from meal ☐ Have desire for sweets ☐ Feel hungry again soon after meal ☐ Need to snack between meals
ENERGY LEVELS	Normal energy response to meal: ☐ Energy is restored after eating ☐ Have good, lasting, "normal" sense of energy and well-being	Poor energy response to meal: ☐ Too much or too little energy ☐ Become hyper, jittery, shaky, nervous, or speedy ☐ Feel hyper, but exhausted "underneath" ☐ Energy drop, fatigue, exhaustion, sleepiness, drowsiness, lethargy, or listlessness
MENTAL EMOTIONAL WELL-BEING	Normal qualities: ☐ Improved well-being ☐ Sense of feeling refueled and restored ☐ Upliftment in emotions ☐ Improved clarity and acuity of mind ☐ Normalization of thought processes	Abnormal qualities: ☐ Mentally slow, sluggish, spacey ☐ Inability to think quickly or clearly ☐ Hyper, overly rapid thoughts ☐ Inability to focus/hold attention ☐ Hypo traits: Apathy, depression, sadness ☐ Hyper traits: Anxious, obsessive, fearful, angry, short tempered, or irritable, etc.

DIET AND EXERCISE JOURNAL   WEEK 3 / DAY 15

Date : _____

Diet and Exercise Goals : _____

_____

_____

_____

_____

Meal	List of Food You Ate	Additional Notes
Breakfast		
Lunch		
Dinner		
Snack		

	Exercises	Duration, Repetitions and Additional Notes
Body Balancing Streches		
Core Stability Exercises		
Body Allignment Exercises		

Do what you can, with what you have, where you are. - Theodore Roosevelt

Diet Record Sheet	☐Breakfast ☐Lunch ☐Dinner	
Reactions after a meal	**Good**	**Bad**
APPETITE FULLNESS / SATISFACTION SWEET CRAVINGS	Following the meal . . . ☐ Feel full, satisfied ☐ Do NOT have sweet cravings ☐ Do NOT desire more food ☐ Do NOT get hungry soon after ☐ Do NOT need to snack before next meal	Following the meal . . . ☐ Feel physically full, but still hungry ☐ Don't feel satisfied; feel like something was missing from meal ☐ Have desire for sweets ☐ Feel hungry again soon after meal ☐ Need to snack between meals
ENERGY LEVELS	Normal energy response to meal: ☐ Energy is restored after eating ☐ Have good, lasting, "normal" sense of energy and well-being	Poor energy response to meal: ☐ Too much or too little energy ☐ Become hyper, jittery, shaky, nervous, or speedy ☐ Feel hyper, but exhausted "underneath" ☐ Energy drop, fatigue, exhaustion, sleepiness, drowsiness, lethargy, or listlessness
MENTAL EMOTIONAL WELL-BEING	Normal qualities: ☐ Improved well-being ☐ Sense of feeling refueled and restored ☐ Upliftment in emotions ☐ Improved clarity and acuity of mind ☐ Normalization of thought processes	Abnormal qualities: ☐ Mentally slow, sluggish, spacey ☐ Inability to think quickly or clearly ☐ Hyper, overly rapid thoughts ☐ Inability to focus/hold attention ☐ Hypo traits: Apathy, depression, sadness ☐ Hyper traits: Anxious, obsessive, fearful, angry, short tempered, or irritable, etc.

DIET AND EXERCISE JOURNAL   WEEK 3 / DAY 16

Date : _____

Diet and Exercise Goals : _____

_____

_____

_____

_____

Meal	List of Food You Ate	Additional Notes
Breakfast		
Lunch		
Dinner		
Snack		

	Exercises	Duration, Repetitions and Additional Notes
Body Balancing Streches		
Core Stability Exercises		
Body Allignment Exercises		

Everything you can imagine is real. - Pablo Picasso

Diet Record Sheet	☐Breakfast ☐Lunch ☐Dinner	
Reactions after a meal	Good	Bad
APPETITE FULLNESS / SATISFACTION SWEET CRAVINGS	Following the meal . . . ☐ Feel full, satisfied ☐ Do NOT have sweet cravings ☐ Do NOT desire more food ☐ Do NOT get hungry soon after ☐ Do NOT need to snack before next meal	Following the meal . . . ☐ Feel physically full, but still hungry ☐ Don't feel satisfied; feel like something was missing from meal ☐ Have desire for sweets ☐ Feel hungry again soon after meal ☐ Need to snack between meals
ENERGY LEVELS	Normal energy response to meal: ☐ Energy is restored after eating ☐ Have good, lasting, "normal" sense of energy and well-being	Poor energy response to meal: ☐ Too much or too little energy ☐ Become hyper, jittery, shaky, nervous, or speedy ☐ Feel hyper, but exhausted "underneath" ☐ Energy drop, fatigue, exhaustion, sleepiness, drowsiness, lethargy, or listlessness
MENTAL EMOTIONAL WELL-BEING	Normal qualities: ☐ Improved well-being ☐ Sense of feeling refueled and restored ☐ Upliftment in emotions ☐ Improved clarity and acuity of mind ☐ Normalization of thought processes	Abnormal qualities: ☐ Mentally slow, sluggish, spacey ☐ Inability to think quickly or clearly ☐ Hyper, overly rapid thoughts ☐ Inability to focus/hold attention ☐ Hypo traits: Apathy, depression, sadness ☐ Hyper traits: Anxious, obsessive, fearful, angry, short tempered, or irritable, etc.

DIET AND EXERCISE JOURNAL   WEEK 3 / DAY 17

Date : _____

Diet and Exercise Goals : _____

_____

_____

_____

_____

Meal	List of Food You Ate	Additional Notes
Breakfast		
Lunch		
Dinner		
Snack		

	Exercises	Duration, Repetitions and Additional Notes
Body Balancing Streches		
Core Stability Exercises		
Body Allignment Exercises		

Maybe everyone can live beyond what they're capable of. - Markus Zusak

Diet Record Sheet	☐Breakfast ☐Lunch ☐Dinner	
Reactions after a meal	Good	Bad
APPETITE FULLNESS / SATISFACTION SWEET CRAVINGS	Following the meal . . . ☐ Feel full, satisfied ☐ Do NOT have sweet cravings ☐ Do NOT desire more food ☐ Do NOT get hungry soon after ☐ Do NOT need to snack before next meal	Following the meal . . . ☐ Feel physically full, but still hungry ☐ Don't feel satisfied; feel like something was missing from meal ☐ Have desire for sweets ☐ Feel hungry again soon after meal ☐ Need to snack between meals
ENERGY LEVELS	Normal energy response to meal: ☐ Energy is restored after eating ☐ Have good, lasting, "normal" sense of energy and well-being	Poor energy response to meal: ☐ Too much or too little energy ☐ Become hyper, jittery, shaky, nervous, or speedy ☐ Feel hyper, but exhausted "underneath" ☐ Energy drop, fatigue, exhaustion, sleepiness, drowsiness, lethargy, or listlessness
MENTAL EMOTIONAL WELL-BEING	Normal qualities: ☐ Improved well-being ☐ Sense of feeling refueled and restored ☐ Upliftment in emotions ☐ Improved clarity and acuity of mind ☐ Normalization of thought processes	Abnormal qualities: ☐ Mentally slow, sluggish, spacey ☐ Inability to think quickly or clearly ☐ Hyper, overly rapid thoughts ☐ Inability to focus/hold attention ☐ Hypo traits: Apathy, depression, sadness ☐ Hyper traits: Anxious, obsessive, fearful, angry, short tempered, or irritable, etc.

DIET AND EXERCISE JOURNAL   WEEK 3 / DAY 18

Date : _____

Diet and Exercise Goals : _____

_____

_____

_____

_____

Meal	List of Food You Ate	Additional Notes
Breakfast		
Lunch		
Dinner		
Snack		

	Exercises	Duration, Repetitions and Additional Notes
Body Balancing Streches		
Core Stability Exercises		
Body Allignment Exercises		

The past has no power over the present moment. - Eckhart Tolle

Diet Record Sheet	☐Breakfast ☐Lunch ☐Dinner	
Reactions after a meal	Good	Bad
APPETITE FULLNESS / SATISFACTION SWEET CRAVINGS	Following the meal . . . ☐ Feel full, satisfied ☐ Do NOT have sweet cravings ☐ Do NOT desire more food ☐ Do NOT get hungry soon after ☐ Do NOT need to snack before next meal	Following the meal . . . ☐ Feel physically full, but still hungry ☐ Don't feel satisfied; feel like something was missing from meal ☐ Have desire for sweets ☐ Feel hungry again soon after meal ☐ Need to snack between meals
ENERGY LEVELS	Normal energy response to meal: ☐ Energy is restored after eating ☐ Have good, lasting, "normal" sense of energy and well-being	Poor energy response to meal: ☐ Too much or too little energy ☐ Become hyper, jittery, shaky, nervous, or speedy ☐ Feel hyper, but exhausted "underneath" ☐ Energy drop, fatigue, exhaustion, sleepiness, drowsiness, lethargy, or listlessness
MENTAL EMOTIONAL WELL-BEING	Normal qualities: ☐ Improved well-being ☐ Sense of feeling refueled and restored ☐ Upliftment in emotions ☐ Improved clarity and acuity of mind ☐ Normalization of thought processes	Abnormal qualities: ☐ Mentally slow, sluggish, spacey ☐ Inability to think quickly or clearly ☐ Hyper, overly rapid thoughts ☐ Inability to focus/hold attention ☐ Hypo traits: Apathy, depression, sadness ☐ Hyper traits: Anxious, obsessive, fearful, angry, short tempered, or irritable, etc.

DIET AND EXERCISE JOURNAL   WEEK 3 / DAY 19

Date : _____

Diet and Exercise Goals : _____

_____

_____

_____

_____

_____

Meal	List of Food You Ate	Additional Notes
Breakfast		
Lunch		
Dinner		
Snack		

	Exercises	Duration, Repetitions and Additional Notes
Body Balancing Streches		
Core Stability Exercises		
Body Allignment Exercises		

I started my life with a single absolute: that the world was mine to shape in the image of my highest values and never to be given up to a lesser standard, no matter how long or hard the struggle. - Ayn Rand

Diet Record Sheet	☐Breakfast ☐Lunch ☐Dinner	
Reactions after a meal	Good	Bad
APPETITE FULLNESS / SATISFACTION SWEET CRAVINGS	Following the meal . . . ☐ Feel full, satisfied ☐ Do NOT have sweet cravings ☐ Do NOT desire more food ☐ Do NOT get hungry soon after ☐ Do NOT need to snack before next meal	Following the meal . . . ☐ Feel physically full, but still hungry ☐ Don't feel satisfied; feel like something was missing from meal ☐ Have desire for sweets ☐ Feel hungry again soon after meal ☐ Need to snack between meals
ENERGY LEVELS	Normal energy response to meal: ☐ Energy is restored after eating ☐ Have good, lasting, "normal" sense of energy and well-being	Poor energy response to meal: ☐ Too much or too little energy ☐ Become hyper, jittery, shaky, nervous, or speedy ☐ Feel hyper, but exhausted "underneath" ☐ Energy drop, fatigue, exhaustion, sleepiness, drowsiness, lethargy, or listlessness
MENTAL EMOTIONAL WELL-BEING	Normal qualities: ☐ Improved well-being ☐ Sense of feeling refueled and restored ☐ Upliftment in emotions ☐ Improved clarity and acuity of mind ☐ Normalization of thought processes	Abnormal qualities: ☐ Mentally slow, sluggish, spacey ☐ Inability to think quickly or clearly ☐ Hyper, overly rapid thoughts ☐ Inability to focus/hold attention ☐ Hypo traits: Apathy, depression, sadness ☐ Hyper traits: Anxious, obsessive, fearful, angry, short tempered, or irritable, etc.

DIET AND EXERCISE JOURNAL   WEEK 3 / DAY 20

Date : _____

Diet and Exercise Goals : _____

_____

_____

_____

_____

Meal	List of Food You Ate	Additional Notes
Breakfast		
Lunch		
Dinner		
Snack		

	Exercises	Duration, Repetitions and Additional Notes
Body Balancing Streches		
Core Stability Exercises		
Body Allignment Exercises		

Trust yourself. You know more than you think you do. - Benjamin Spock

Diet Record Sheet	☐Breakfast	☐Lunch	☐Dinner

Reactions after a meal	Good	Bad
APPETITE FULLNESS / SATISFACTION SWEET CRAVINGS	Following the meal . . . ☐ Feel full, satisfied ☐ Do NOT have sweet cravings ☐ Do NOT desire more food ☐ Do NOT get hungry soon after ☐ Do NOT need to snack before next meal	Following the meal . . . ☐ Feel physically full, but still hungry ☐ Don't feel satisfied; feel like something was missing from meal ☐ Have desire for sweets ☐ Feel hungry again soon after meal ☐ Need to snack between meals
ENERGY LEVELS	Normal energy response to meal: ☐ Energy is restored after eating ☐ Have good, lasting, "normal" sense of energy and well-being	Poor energy response to meal: ☐ Too much or too little energy ☐ Become hyper, jittery, shaky, nervous, or speedy ☐ Feel hyper, but exhausted "underneath" ☐ Energy drop, fatigue, exhaustion, sleepiness, drowsiness, lethargy, or listlessness
MENTAL EMOTIONAL WELL-BEING	Normal qualities: ☐ Improved well-being ☐ Sense of feeling refueled and restored ☐ Upliftment in emotions ☐ Improved clarity and acuity of mind ☐ Normalization of thought processes	Abnormal qualities: ☐ Mentally slow, sluggish, spacey ☐ Inability to think quickly or clearly ☐ Hyper, overly rapid thoughts ☐ Inability to focus/hold attention ☐ Hypo traits: Apathy, depression, sadness ☐ Hyper traits: Anxious, obsessive, fearful, angry, short tempered, or irritable, etc.

DIET AND EXERCISE JOURNAL   WEEK 3 / DAY 21

Date : _____

Diet and Exercise Goals : _____

_____

_____

_____

_____

Meal	List of Food You Ate	Additional Notes
Breakfast		
Lunch		
Dinner		
Snack		

	Exercises	Duration, Repetitions and Additional Notes
Body Balancing Streches		
Core Stability Exercises		
Body Allignment Exercises		

Don't cry because it's over, smile because it happened. - Dr. Seuss

Diet Record Sheet	☐ Breakfast ☐ Lunch ☐ Dinner	
Reactions after a meal	**Good**	**Bad**
APPETITE FULLNESS / SATISFACTION SWEET CRAVINGS	Following the meal . . . ☐ Feel full, satisfied ☐ Do NOT have sweet cravings ☐ Do NOT desire more food ☐ Do NOT get hungry soon after ☐ Do NOT need to snack before next meal	Following the meal . . . ☐ Feel physically full, but still hungry ☐ Don't feel satisfied; feel like something was missing from meal ☐ Have desire for sweets ☐ Feel hungry again soon after meal ☐ Need to snack between meals
ENERGY LEVELS	Normal energy response to meal: ☐ Energy is restored after eating ☐ Have good, lasting, "normal" sense of energy and well-being	Poor energy response to meal: ☐ Too much or too little energy ☐ Become hyper, jittery, shaky, nervous, or speedy ☐ Feel hyper, but exhausted "underneath" ☐ Energy drop, fatigue, exhaustion, sleepiness, drowsiness, lethargy, or listlessness
MENTAL EMOTIONAL WELL-BEING	Normal qualities: ☐ Improved well-being ☐ Sense of feeling refueled and restored ☐ Upliftment in emotions ☐ Improved clarity and acuity of mind ☐ Normalization of thought processes	Abnormal qualities: ☐ Mentally slow, sluggish, spacey ☐ Inability to think quickly or clearly ☐ Hyper, overly rapid thoughts ☐ Inability to focus/hold attention ☐ Hypo traits: Apathy, depression, sadness ☐ Hyper traits: Anxious, obsessive, fearful, angry, short tempered, or irritable, etc.

Week 4: Scoliosis Symptoms Review

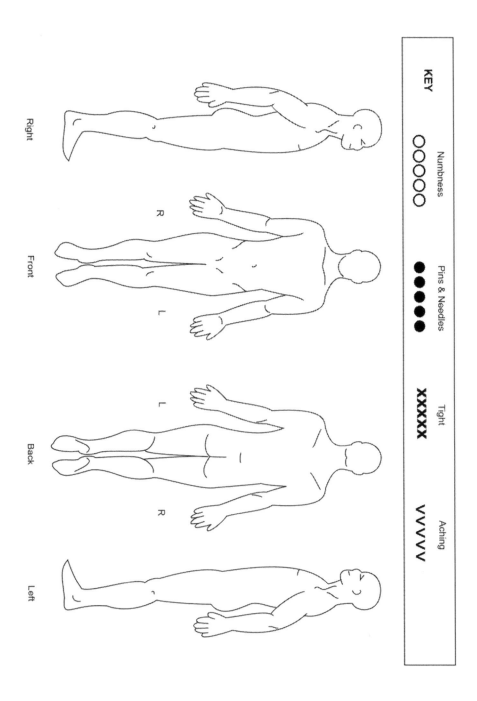

Week 4: Trigger Point Mapping

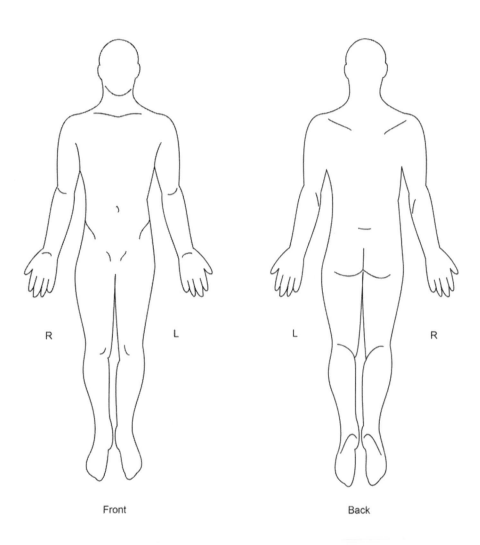

R   L   L   R

Front   Back

DIET AND EXERCISE JOURNAL   WEEK 4 / DAY 22

Date : _____

Diet and Exercise Goals : _____

_____

_____

_____

_____

Meal	List of Food You Ate	Additional Notes
Breakfast		
Lunch		
Dinner		
Snack		

	Exercises	Duration, Repetitions and Additional Notes
Body Balancing Streches		
Core Stability Exercises		
Body Allignment Exercises		

I can't change the direction of the wind,
but I can adjust my sails to always reach my destination. - Jimmy Dean

Diet Record Sheet	☐Breakfast ☐Lunch ☐Dinner	
Reactions after a meal	**Good**	**Bad**
APPETITE FULLNESS / SATISFACTION SWEET CRAVINGS	Following the meal . . . ☐ Feel full, satisfied ☐ Do NOT have sweet cravings ☐ Do NOT desire more food ☐ Do NOT get hungry soon after ☐ Do NOT need to snack before next meal	Following the meal . . . ☐ Feel physically full, but still hungry ☐ Don't feel satisfied; feel like something was missing from meal ☐ Have desire for sweets ☐ Feel hungry again soon after meal ☐ Need to snack between meals
ENERGY LEVELS	Normal energy response to meal: ☐ Energy is restored after eating ☐ Have good, lasting, "normal" sense of energy and well-being	Poor energy response to meal: ☐ Too much or too little energy ☐ Become hyper, jittery, shaky, nervous, or speedy ☐ Feel hyper, but exhausted "underneath" ☐ Energy drop, fatigue, exhaustion, sleepiness, drowsiness, lethargy, or listlessness
MENTAL EMOTIONAL WELL-BEING	Normal qualities: ☐ Improved well-being ☐ Sense of feeling refueled and restored ☐ Upliftment in emotions ☐ Improved clarity and acuity of mind ☐ Normalization of thought processes	Abnormal qualities: ☐ Mentally slow, sluggish, spacey ☐ Inability to think quickly or clearly ☐ Hyper, overly rapid thoughts ☐ Inability to focus/hold attention ☐ Hypo traits: Apathy, depression, sadness ☐ Hyper traits: Anxious, obsessive, fearful, angry, short tempered, or irritable, etc.

DIET AND EXERCISE JOURNAL   WEEK 4 / DAY 23

Date : _____

Diet and Exercise Goals : _____

_____

_____

_____

_____

Meal	List of Food You Ate	Additional Notes
Breakfast		
Lunch		
Dinner		
Snack		

	Exercises	Duration, Repetitions and Additional Notes
Body Balancing Streches		
Core Stability Exercises		
Body Allignment Exercises		

We can change our lives. We can do, have, and be exactly what we wish. - Tony Robbins

Diet Record Sheet	☐Breakfast ☐Lunch ☐Dinner	
Reactions after a meal	**Good**	**Bad**
APPETITE FULLNESS / SATISFACTION SWEET CRAVINGS	Following the meal . . . ☐ Feel full, satisfied ☐ Do NOT have sweet cravings ☐ Do NOT desire more food ☐ Do NOT get hungry soon after ☐ Do NOT need to snack before next meal	Following the meal . . . ☐ Feel physically full, but still hungry ☐ Don't feel satisfied; feel like something was missing from meal ☐ Have desire for sweets ☐ Feel hungry again soon after meal ☐ Need to snack between meals
ENERGY LEVELS	Normal energy response to meal: ☐ Energy is restored after eating ☐ Have good, lasting, "normal" sense of energy and well-being	Poor energy response to meal: ☐ Too much or too little energy ☐ Become hyper, jittery, shaky, nervous, or speedy ☐ Feel hyper, but exhausted "underneath" ☐ Energy drop, fatigue, exhaustion, sleepiness, drowsiness, lethargy, or listlessness
MENTAL EMOTIONAL WELL-BEING	Normal qualities: ☐ Improved well-being ☐ Sense of feeling refueled and restored ☐ Upliftment in emotions ☐ Improved clarity and acuity of mind ☐ Normalization of thought processes	Abnormal qualities: ☐ Mentally slow, sluggish, spacey ☐ Inability to think quickly or clearly ☐ Hyper, overly rapid thoughts ☐ Inability to focus/hold attention ☐ Hypo traits: Apathy, depression, sadness ☐ Hyper traits: Anxious, obsessive, fearful, angry, short tempered, or irritable, etc.

DIET AND EXERCISE JOURNAL

WEEK 4 / DAY 24

Date : _____

Diet and Exercise Goals : _____

_____

_____

_____

_____

_____

Meal	List of Food You Ate	Additional Notes
Breakfast		
Lunch		
Dinner		
Snack		

	Exercises	Duration, Repetitions and Additional Notes
Body Balancing Streches		
Core Stability Exercises		
Body Allignment Exercises		

It is by acts and not by ideas that people live. - Harry Emerson Fosdick

Diet Record Sheet	☐Breakfast ☐Lunch ☐Dinner	
Reactions after a meal	**Good**	**Bad**
APPETITE FULLNESS / SATISFACTION SWEET CRAVINGS	Following the meal . . . ☐ Feel full, satisfied ☐ Do NOT have sweet cravings ☐ Do NOT desire more food ☐ Do NOT get hungry soon after ☐ Do NOT need to snack before next meal	Following the meal . . . ☐ Feel physically full, but still hungry ☐ Don't feel satisfied; feel like something was missing from meal ☐ Have desire for sweets ☐ Feel hungry again soon after meal ☐ Need to snack between meals
ENERGY LEVELS	Normal energy response to meal: ☐ Energy is restored after eating ☐ Have good, lasting, "normal" sense of energy and well-being	Poor energy response to meal: ☐ Too much or too little energy ☐ Become hyper, jittery, shaky, nervous, or speedy ☐ Feel hyper, but exhausted "underneath" ☐ Energy drop, fatigue, exhaustion, sleepiness, drowsiness, lethargy, or listlessness
MENTAL EMOTIONAL WELL-BEING	Normal qualities: ☐ Improved well-being ☐ Sense of feeling refueled and restored ☐ Upliftment in emotions ☐ Improved clarity and acuity of mind ☐ Normalization of thought processes	Abnormal qualities: ☐ Mentally slow, sluggish, spacey ☐ Inability to think quickly or clearly ☐ Hyper, overly rapid thoughts ☐ Inability to focus/hold attention ☐ Hypo traits: Apathy, depression, sadness ☐ Hyper traits: Anxious, obsessive, fearful, angry, short tempered, or irritable, etc.

DIET AND EXERCISE JOURNAL   WEEK 4 / DAY 25

Date : _____

Diet and Exercise Goals : _____

_____

_____

_____

_____

Meal	List of Food You Ate	Additional Notes
Breakfast		
Lunch		
Dinner		
Snack		

	Exercises	Duration, Repetitions and Additional Notes
Body Balancing Streches		
Core Stability Exercises		
Body Allignment Exercises		

You are always free to change your mind and choose a different future, or a different past. - Richard Bach

Diet Record Sheet	☐Breakfast ☐Lunch ☐Dinner	
Reactions after a meal	Good	Bad
APPETITE FULLNESS / SATISFACTION SWEET CRAVINGS	Following the meal . . . ☐ Feel full, satisfied ☐ Do NOT have sweet cravings ☐ Do NOT desire more food ☐ Do NOT get hungry soon after ☐ Do NOT need to snack before next meal	Following the meal . . . ☐ Feel physically full, but still hungry ☐ Don't feel satisfied; feel like something was missing from meal ☐ Have desire for sweets ☐ Feel hungry again soon after meal ☐ Need to snack between meals
ENERGY LEVELS	Normal energy response to meal: ☐ Energy is restored after eating ☐ Have good, lasting, "normal" sense of energy and well-being	Poor energy response to meal: ☐ Too much or too little energy ☐ Become hyper, jittery, shaky, nervous, or speedy ☐ Feel hyper, but exhausted "underneath" ☐ Energy drop, fatigue, exhaustion, sleepiness, drowsiness, lethargy, or listlessness
MENTAL EMOTIONAL WELL-BEING	Normal qualities: ☐ Improved well-being ☐ Sense of feeling refueled and restored ☐ Upliftment in emotions ☐ Improved clarity and acuity of mind ☐ Normalization of thought processes	Abnormal qualities: ☐ Mentally slow, sluggish, spacey ☐ Inability to think quickly or clearly ☐ Hyper, overly rapid thoughts ☐ Inability to focus/hold attention ☐ Hypo traits: Apathy, depression, sadness ☐ Hyper traits: Anxious, obsessive, fearful, angry, short tempered, or irritable, etc.

DIET AND EXERCISE JOURNAL   WEEK 4 / DAY 26

Date : _____

Diet and Exercise Goals : _____

_____

_____

_____

_____

Meal	List of Food You Ate	Additional Notes
Breakfast		
Lunch		
Dinner		
Snack		

	Exercises	Duration, Repetitions and Additional Notes
Body Balancing Streches		
Core Stability Exercises		
Body Allignment Exercises		

Sports do not build character. They reveal it. - Heywood Broun

Diet Record Sheet	☐Breakfast ☐Lunch ☐Dinner	
Reactions after a meal	**Good**	**Bad**
APPETITE FULLNESS / SATISFACTION SWEET CRAVINGS	Following the meal . . . ☐ Feel full, satisfied ☐ Do NOT have sweet cravings ☐ Do NOT desire more food ☐ Do NOT get hungry soon after ☐ Do NOT need to snack before next meal	Following the meal . . . ☐ Feel physically full, but still hungry ☐ Don't feel satisfied; feel like something was missing from meal ☐ Have desire for sweets ☐ Feel hungry again soon after meal ☐ Need to snack between meals
ENERGY LEVELS	Normal energy response to meal: ☐ Energy is restored after eating ☐ Have good, lasting, "normal" sense of energy and well-being	Poor energy response to meal: ☐ Too much or too little energy ☐ Become hyper, jittery, shaky, nervous, or speedy ☐ Feel hyper, but exhausted "underneath" ☐ Energy drop, fatigue, exhaustion, sleepiness, drowsiness, lethargy, or listlessness
MENTAL EMOTIONAL WELL-BEING	Normal qualities: ☐ Improved well-being ☐ Sense of feeling refueled and restored ☐ Upliftment in emotions ☐ Improved clarity and acuity of mind ☐ Normalization of thought processes	Abnormal qualities: ☐ Mentally slow, sluggish, spacey ☐ Inability to think quickly or clearly ☐ Hyper, overly rapid thoughts ☐ Inability to focus/hold attention ☐ Hypo traits: Apathy, depression, sadness ☐ Hyper traits: Anxious, obsessive, fearful, angry, short tempered, or irritable, etc.

DIET AND EXERCISE JOURNAL   WEEK 4 / DAY 27

Date : _____

Diet and Exercise Goals : _____

_____

_____

_____

_____

Meal	List of Food You Ate	Additional Notes
Breakfast		
Lunch		
Dinner		
Snack		

	Exercises	Duration, Repetitions and Additional Notes
Body Balancing Streches		
Core Stability Exercises		
Body Allignment Exercises		

If you don't like something, change it. If you can't change it, change your attitude. - Maya Angelou

Diet Record Sheet		☐Breakfast ☐Lunch ☐Dinner
Reactions after a meal	Good	Bad
APPETITE FULLNESS / SATISFACTION SWEET CRAVINGS	Following the meal . . . ☐ Feel full, satisfied ☐ Do NOT have sweet cravings ☐ Do NOT desire more food ☐ Do NOT get hungry soon after ☐ Do NOT need to snack before next meal	Following the meal . . . ☐ Feel physically full, but still hungry ☐ Don't feel satisfied; feel like something was missing from meal ☐ Have desire for sweets ☐ Feel hungry again soon after meal ☐ Need to snack between meals
ENERGY LEVELS	Normal energy response to meal: ☐ Energy is restored after eating ☐ Have good, lasting, "normal" sense of energy and well-being	Poor energy response to meal: ☐ Too much or too little energy ☐ Become hyper, jittery, shaky, nervous, or speedy ☐ Feel hyper, but exhausted "underneath" ☐ Energy drop, fatigue, exhaustion, sleepiness, drowsiness, lethargy, or listlessness
MENTAL EMOTIONAL WELL-BEING	Normal qualities: ☐ Improved well-being ☐ Sense of feeling refueled and restored ☐ Upliftment in emotions ☐ Improved clarity and acuity of mind ☐ Normalization of thought processes	Abnormal qualities: ☐ Mentally slow, sluggish, spacey ☐ Inability to think quickly or clearly ☐ Hyper, overly rapid thoughts ☐ Inability to focus/hold attention ☐ Hypo traits: Apathy, depression, sadness ☐ Hyper traits: Anxious, obsessive, fearful, angry, short tempered, or irritable, etc.

DIET AND EXERCISE JOURNAL   WEEK 4 / DAY 28

Date : _____

Diet and Exercise Goals : _____

_____

_____

_____

_____

Meal	List of Food You Ate	Additional Notes
Breakfast		
Lunch		
Dinner		
Snack		

	Exercises	Duration, Repetitions and Additional Notes
Body Balancing Streches		
Core Stability Exercises		
Body Allignment Exercises		

Everyone thinks of changing the world, but no one thinks of changing himself. - Leo Tolstoy

Diet Record Sheet	☐Breakfast ☐Lunch ☐Dinner	
Reactions after a meal	**Good**	**Bad**
APPETITE FULLNESS / SATISFACTION SWEET CRAVINGS	Following the meal . . . ☐ Feel full, satisfied ☐ Do NOT have sweet cravings ☐ Do NOT desire more food ☐ Do NOT get hungry soon after ☐ Do NOT need to snack before next meal	Following the meal . . . ☐ Feel physically full, but still hungry ☐ Don't feel satisfied; feel like something was missing from meal ☐ Have desire for sweets ☐ Feel hungry again soon after meal ☐ Need to snack between meals
ENERGY LEVELS	Normal energy response to meal: ☐ Energy is restored after eating ☐ Have good, lasting, "normal" sense of energy and well-being	Poor energy response to meal: ☐ Too much or too little energy ☐ Become hyper, jittery, shaky, nervous, or speedy ☐ Feel hyper, but exhausted "underneath" ☐ Energy drop, fatigue, exhaustion, sleepiness, drowsiness, lethargy, or listlessness
MENTAL EMOTIONAL WELL-BEING	Normal qualities: ☐ Improved well-being ☐ Sense of feeling refueled and restored ☐ Upliftment in emotions ☐ Improved clarity and acuity of mind ☐ Normalization of thought processes	Abnormal qualities: ☐ Mentally slow, sluggish, spacey ☐ Inability to think quickly or clearly ☐ Hyper, overly rapid thoughts ☐ Inability to focus/hold attention ☐ Hypo traits: Apathy, depression, sadness ☐ Hyper traits: Anxious, obsessive, fearful, angry, short tempered, or irritable, etc.

DIET AND EXERCISE JOURNAL

WEEK 5 / DAY 29

Date : _____

Diet and Exercise Goals : _____

_____

_____

_____

_____

Meal	List of Food You Ate	Additional Notes
Breakfast		
Lunch		
Dinner		
Snack		

	Exercises	Duration, Repetitions and Additional Notes
Body Balancing Streches		
Core Stability Exercises		
Body Allignment Exercises		

If we don't change, we don't grow. If we don't grow, we aren't really living. - Gail Sheehy

Diet Record Sheet	☐Breakfast ☐Lunch ☐Dinner	
Reactions after a meal	Good	Bad
APPETITE FULLNESS / SATISFACTION SWEET CRAVINGS	Following the meal . . . ☐ Feel full, satisfied ☐ Do NOT have sweet cravings ☐ Do NOT desire more food ☐ Do NOT get hungry soon after ☐ Do NOT need to snack before next meal	Following the meal . . . ☐ Feel physically full, but still hungry ☐ Don't feel satisfied; feel like something was missing from meal ☐ Have desire for sweets ☐ Feel hungry again soon after meal ☐ Need to snack between meals
ENERGY LEVELS	Normal energy response to meal: ☐ Energy is restored after eating ☐ Have good, lasting, "normal" sense of energy and well-being	Poor energy response to meal: ☐ Too much or too little energy ☐ Become hyper, jittery, shaky, nervous, or speedy ☐ Feel hyper, but exhausted "underneath" ☐ Energy drop, fatigue, exhaustion, sleepiness, drowsiness, lethargy, or listlessness
MENTAL EMOTIONAL WELL-BEING	Normal qualities: ☐ Improved well-being ☐ Sense of feeling refueled and restored ☐ Upliftment in emotions ☐ Improved clarity and acuity of mind ☐ Normalization of thought processes	Abnormal qualities: ☐ Mentally slow, sluggish, spacey ☐ Inability to think quickly or clearly ☐ Hyper, overly rapid thoughts ☐ Inability to focus/hold attention ☐ Hypo traits: Apathy, depression, sadness ☐ Hyper traits: Anxious, obsessive, fearful, angry, short tempered, or irritable, etc.

DIET AND EXERCISE JOURNAL   WEEK 5 / DAY 30

Date : _____

Diet and Exercise Goals : _____

_____

_____

_____

_____

Meal	List of Food You Ate	Additional Notes
Breakfast		
Lunch		
Dinner		
Snack		

	Exercises	Duration, Repetitions and Additional Notes
Body Balancing Streches		
Core Stability Exercises		
Body Allignment Exercises		

Things do not change; we change. - Henry David Thoreau

Diet Record Sheet		☐Breakfast　☐Lunch　☐Dinner
Reactions after a meal	**Good**	**Bad**
APPETITE FULLNESS / SATISFACTION SWEET CRAVINGS	Following the meal . . . ☐ Feel full, satisfied ☐ Do NOT have sweet cravings ☐ Do NOT desire more food ☐ Do NOT get hungry soon after ☐ Do NOT need to snack before next meal	Following the meal . . . ☐ Feel physically full, but still hungry ☐ Don't feel satisfied; feel like something was missing from meal ☐ Have desire for sweets ☐ Feel hungry again soon after meal ☐ Need to snack between meals
ENERGY LEVELS	Normal energy response to meal: ☐ Energy is restored after eating ☐ Have good, lasting, "normal" sense of energy and well-being	Poor energy response to meal: ☐ Too much or too little energy ☐ Become hyper, jittery, shaky, nervous, or speedy ☐ Feel hyper, but exhausted "underneath" ☐ Energy drop, fatigue, exhaustion, sleepiness, drowsiness, lethargy, or listlessness
MENTAL EMOTIONAL WELL-BEING	Normal qualities: ☐ Improved well-being ☐ Sense of feeling refueled and restored ☐ Upliftment in emotions ☐ Improved clarity and acuity of mind ☐ Normalization of thought processes	Abnormal qualities: ☐ Mentally slow, sluggish, spacey ☐ Inability to think quickly or clearly ☐ Hyper, overly rapid thoughts ☐ Inability to focus/hold attention ☐ Hypo traits: Apathy, depression, sadness ☐ Hyper traits: Anxious, obsessive, fearful, angry, short tempered, or irritable, etc.

DIET AND EXERCISE JOURNAL　　　　　　　WEEK 5 / DAY 31

Date : _____

Diet and Exercise Goals : _____

_____

_____

_____

_____

Meal	List of Food You Ate	Additional Notes
Breakfast		
Lunch		
Dinner		
Snack		

	Exercises	Duration, Repetitions and Additional Notes
Body Balancing Streches		
Core Stability Exercises		
Body Allignment Exercises		

The only way to finish is to start. - Author Unknown

Diet Record Sheet		☐ Breakfast ☐ Lunch ☐ Dinner
Reactions after a meal	Good	Bad
APPETITE FULLNESS / SATISFACTION SWEET CRAVINGS	Following the meal . . . ☐ Feel full, satisfied ☐ Do NOT have sweet cravings ☐ Do NOT desire more food ☐ Do NOT get hungry soon after ☐ Do NOT need to snack before next meal	Following the meal . . . ☐ Feel physically full, but still hungry ☐ Don't feel satisfied; feel like something was missing from meal ☐ Have desire for sweets ☐ Feel hungry again soon after meal ☐ Need to snack between meals
ENERGY LEVELS	Normal energy response to meal: ☐ Energy is restored after eating ☐ Have good, lasting, "normal" sense of energy and well-being	Poor energy response to meal: ☐ Too much or too little energy ☐ Become hyper, jittery, shaky, nervous, or speedy ☐ Feel hyper, but exhausted "underneath" ☐ Energy drop, fatigue, exhaustion, sleepiness, drowsiness, lethargy, or listlessness
MENTAL EMOTIONAL WELL-BEING	Normal qualities: ☐ Improved well-being ☐ Sense of feeling refueled and restored ☐ Upliftment in emotions ☐ Improved clarity and acuity of mind ☐ Normalization of thought processes	Abnormal qualities: ☐ Mentally slow, sluggish, spacey ☐ Inability to think quickly or clearly ☐ Hyper, overly rapid thoughts ☐ Inability to focus/hold attention ☐ Hypo traits: Apathy, depression, sadness ☐ Hyper traits: Anxious, obsessive, fearful, angry, short tempered, or irritable, etc.

DIET AND EXERCISE JOURNAL   WEEK 5 / DAY 32

Date : _____

Diet and Exercise Goals : _____

_____

_____

_____

_____

Meal	List of Food You Ate	Additional Notes
Breakfast		
Lunch		
Dinner		
Snack		

	Exercises	Duration, Repetitions and Additional Notes
Body Balancing Streches		
Core Stability Exercises		
Body Allignment Exercises		

In order to succeed, your desire for success should be greater than your fear of failure. - Bill Cosby

Diet Record Sheet	☐Breakfast ☐Lunch ☐Dinner	
Reactions after a meal	**Good**	**Bad**
APPETITE FULLNESS / SATISFACTION SWEET CRAVINGS	Following the meal . . . ☐ Feel full, satisfied ☐ Do NOT have sweet cravings ☐ Do NOT desire more food ☐ Do NOT get hungry soon after ☐ Do NOT need to snack before next meal	Following the meal . . . ☐ Feel physically full, but still hungry ☐ Don't feel satisfied; feel like something was missing from meal ☐ Have desire for sweets ☐ Feel hungry again soon after meal ☐ Need to snack between meals
ENERGY LEVELS	Normal energy response to meal: ☐ Energy is restored after eating ☐ Have good, lasting, "normal" sense of energy and well-being	Poor energy response to meal: ☐ Too much or too little energy ☐ Become hyper, jittery, shaky, nervous, or speedy ☐ Feel hyper, but exhausted "underneath" ☐ Energy drop, fatigue, exhaustion, sleepiness, drowsiness, lethargy, or listlessness
MENTAL EMOTIONAL WELL-BEING	Normal qualities: ☐ Improved well-being ☐ Sense of feeling refueled and restored ☐ Upliftment in emotions ☐ Improved clarity and acuity of mind ☐ Normalization of thought processes	Abnormal qualities: ☐ Mentally slow, sluggish, spacey ☐ Inability to think quickly or clearly ☐ Hyper, overly rapid thoughts ☐ Inability to focus/hold attention ☐ Hypo traits: Apathy, depression, sadness ☐ Hyper traits: Anxious, obsessive, fearful, angry, short tempered, or irritable, etc.

DIET AND EXERCISE JOURNAL   WEEK 5 / DAY 33

Date : _____

Diet and Exercise Goals : _____

_____

_____

_____

_____

Meal	List of Food You Ate	Additional Notes
Breakfast		
Lunch		
Dinner		
Snack		

	Exercises	Duration, Repetitions and Additional Notes
Body Balancing Streches		
Core Stability Exercises		
Body Allignment Exercises		

The will to win, the desire to succeed, the urge to reach your full potential...
these are the keys that will unlock the door to personal excellence. – Confucius

Diet Record Sheet	☐Breakfast ☐Lunch ☐Dinner	
Reactions after a meal	**Good**	**Bad**
APPETITE FULLNESS / SATISFACTION SWEET CRAVINGS	Following the meal . . . ☐ Feel full, satisfied ☐ Do NOT have sweet cravings ☐ Do NOT desire more food ☐ Do NOT get hungry soon after ☐ Do NOT need to snack before next meal	Following the meal . . . ☐ Feel physically full, but still hungry ☐ Don't feel satisfied; feel like something was missing from meal ☐ Have desire for sweets ☐ Feel hungry again soon after meal ☐ Need to snack between meals
ENERGY LEVELS	Normal energy response to meal: ☐ Energy is restored after eating ☐ Have good, lasting, "normal" sense of energy and well-being	Poor energy response to meal: ☐ Too much or too little energy ☐ Become hyper, jittery, shaky, nervous, or speedy ☐ Feel hyper, but exhausted "underneath" ☐ Energy drop, fatigue, exhaustion, sleepiness, drowsiness, lethargy, or listlessness
MENTAL EMOTIONAL WELL-BEING	Normal qualities: ☐ Improved well-being ☐ Sense of feeling refueled and restored ☐ Upliftment in emotions ☐ Improved clarity and acuity of mind ☐ Normalization of thought processes	Abnormal qualities: ☐ Mentally slow, sluggish, spacey ☐ Inability to think quickly or clearly ☐ Hyper, overly rapid thoughts ☐ Inability to focus/hold attention ☐ Hypo traits: Apathy, depression, sadness ☐ Hyper traits: Anxious, obsessive, fearful, angry, short tempered, or irritable, etc.

DIET AND EXERCISE JOURNAL   WEEK 5 / DAY 34

Date : _____

Diet and Exercise Goals : _____

_____

_____

_____

_____

_____

Meal	List of Food You Ate	Additional Notes
Breakfast		
Lunch		
Dinner		
Snack		

	Exercises	Duration, Repetitions and Additional Notes
Body Balancing Streches		
Core Stability Exercises		
Body Allignment Exercises		

The scariest moment is always just before you start. - Stephen King

Diet Record Sheet	☐Breakfast ☐Lunch ☐Dinner	
Reactions after a meal	**Good**	**Bad**
APPETITE FULLNESS / SATISFACTION SWEET CRAVINGS	Following the meal . . . ☐ Feel full, satisfied ☐ Do NOT have sweet cravings ☐ Do NOT desire more food ☐ Do NOT get hungry soon after ☐ Do NOT need to snack before next meal	Following the meal . . . ☐ Feel physically full, but still hungry ☐ Don't feel satisfied; feel like something was missing from meal ☐ Have desire for sweets ☐ Feel hungry again soon after meal ☐ Need to snack between meals
ENERGY LEVELS	Normal energy response to meal: ☐ Energy is restored after eating ☐ Have good, lasting, "normal" sense of energy and well-being	Poor energy response to meal: ☐ Too much or too little energy ☐ Become hyper, jittery, shaky, nervous, or speedy ☐ Feel hyper, but exhausted "underneath" ☐ Energy drop, fatigue, exhaustion, sleepiness, drowsiness, lethargy, or listlessness
MENTAL EMOTIONAL WELL-BEING	Normal qualities: ☐ Improved well-being ☐ Sense of feeling refueled and restored ☐ Upliftment in emotions ☐ Improved clarity and acuity of mind ☐ Normalization of thought processes	Abnormal qualities: ☐ Mentally slow, sluggish, spacey ☐ Inability to think quickly or clearly ☐ Hyper, overly rapid thoughts ☐ Inability to focus/hold attention ☐ Hypo traits: Apathy, depression, sadness ☐ Hyper traits: Anxious, obsessive, fearful, angry, short tempered, or irritable, etc.

DIET AND EXERCISE JOURNAL   WEEK 5 / DAY 35

Date : _____

Diet and Exercise Goals : _____

_____

_____

_____

_____

Meal	List of Food You Ate	Additional Notes
Breakfast		
Lunch		
Dinner		
Snack		

	Exercises	Duration, Repetitions and Additional Notes
Body Balancing Streches		
Core Stability Exercises		
Body Allignment Exercises		

Happy are those who dream dreams and are ready to pay the price
to make them come true. - Leon J. Suenes

Diet Record Sheet	☐Breakfast	☐Lunch	☐Dinner
Reactions after a meal	**Good**	**Bad**	
APPETITE FULLNESS / SATISFACTION SWEET CRAVINGS	Following the meal . . . ☐ Feel full, satisfied ☐ Do NOT have sweet cravings ☐ Do NOT desire more food ☐ Do NOT get hungry soon after ☐ Do NOT need to snack before next meal	Following the meal . . . ☐ Feel physically full, but still hungry ☐ Don't feel satisfied; feel like something was missing from meal ☐ Have desire for sweets ☐ Feel hungry again soon after meal ☐ Need to snack between meals	
ENERGY LEVELS	Normal energy response to meal: ☐ Energy is restored after eating ☐ Have good, lasting, "normal" sense of energy and well-being	Poor energy response to meal: ☐ Too much or too little energy ☐ Become hyper, jittery, shaky, nervous, or speedy ☐ Feel hyper, but exhausted "underneath" ☐ Energy drop, fatigue, exhaustion, sleepiness, drowsiness, lethargy, or listlessness	
MENTAL EMOTIONAL WELL-BEING	Normal qualities: ☐ Improved well-being ☐ Sense of feeling refueled and restored ☐ Upliftment in emotions ☐ Improved clarity and acuity of mind ☐ Normalization of thought processes ´	Abnormal qualities: ☐ Mentally slow, sluggish, spacey ☐ Inability to think quickly or clearly ☐ Hyper, overly rapid thoughts ☐ Inability to focus/hold attention ☐ Hypo traits: Apathy, depression, sadness ☐ Hyper traits: Anxious, obsessive, fearful, angry, short tempered, or irritable, etc.	

DIET AND EXERCISE JOURNAL   WEEK 6 / DAY 36

Date : _____

Diet and Exercise Goals : _____

_____

_____

_____

_____

Meal	List of Food You Ate	Additional Notes
Breakfast		
Lunch		
Dinner		
Snack		

	Exercises	Duration, Repetitions and Additional Notes
Body Balancing Streches		
Core Stability Exercises		
Body Allignment Exercises		

If we are facing in the right direction, all we have to do is keep on walking. - Zen Proverb

Diet Record Sheet	☐ Breakfast ☐ Lunch ☐ Dinner	
Reactions after a meal	**Good**	**Bad**
APPETITE FULLNESS / SATISFACTION SWEET CRAVINGS	Following the meal . . . ☐ Feel full, satisfied ☐ Do NOT have sweet cravings ☐ Do NOT desire more food ☐ Do NOT get hungry soon after ☐ Do NOT need to snack before next meal	Following the meal . . . ☐ Feel physically full, but still hungry ☐ Don't feel satisfied; feel like something was missing from meal ☐ Have desire for sweets ☐ Feel hungry again soon after meal ☐ Need to snack between meals
ENERGY LEVELS	Normal energy response to meal: ☐ Energy is restored after eating ☐ Have good, lasting, "normal" sense of energy and well-being	Poor energy response to meal: ☐ Too much or too little energy ☐ Become hyper, jittery, shaky, nervous, or speedy ☐ Feel hyper, but exhausted "underneath" ☐ Energy drop, fatigue, exhaustion, sleepiness, drowsiness, lethargy, or listlessness
MENTAL EMOTIONAL WELL-BEING	Normal qualities: ☐ Improved well-being ☐ Sense of feeling refueled and restored ☐ Upliftment in emotions ☐ Improved clarity and acuity of mind ☐ Normalization of thought processes	Abnormal qualities: ☐ Mentally slow, sluggish, spacey ☐ Inability to think quickly or clearly ☐ Hyper, overly rapid thoughts ☐ Inability to focus/hold attention ☐ Hypo traits: Apathy, depression, sadness ☐ Hyper traits: Anxious, obsessive, fearful, angry, short tempered, or irritable, etc.

DIET AND EXERCISE JOURNAL   WEEK 6 / DAY 37

Date : _____

Diet and Exercise Goals : _____

_____

_____

_____

_____

Meal	List of Food You Ate	Additional Notes
Breakfast		
Lunch		
Dinner		
Snack		

	Exercises	Duration, Repetitions and Additional Notes
Body Balancing Streches		
Core Stability Exercises		
Body Allignment Exercises		

It is never too late to be what you might have been. - George Eliot

Diet Record Sheet		☐Breakfast ☐Lunch ☐Dinner
Reactions after a meal	**Good**	**Bad**
APPETITE FULLNESS / SATISFACTION SWEET CRAVINGS	Following the meal . . . ☐ Feel full, satisfied ☐ Do NOT have sweet cravings ☐ Do NOT desire more food ☐ Do NOT get hungry soon after ☐ Do NOT need to snack before next meal	Following the meal . . . ☐ Feel physically full, but still hungry ☐ Don't feel satisfied; feel like something was missing from meal ☐ Have desire for sweets ☐ Feel hungry again soon after meal ☐ Need to snack between meals
ENERGY LEVELS	Normal energy response to meal: ☐ Energy is restored after eating ☐ Have good, lasting, "normal" sense of energy and well-being	Poor energy response to meal: ☐ Too much or too little energy ☐ Become hyper, jittery, shaky, nervous, or speedy ☐ Feel hyper, but exhausted "underneath" ☐ Energy drop, fatigue, exhaustion, sleepiness, drowsiness, lethargy, or listlessness
MENTAL EMOTIONAL WELL-BEING	Normal qualities: ☐ Improved well-being ☐ Sense of feeling refueled and restored ☐ Upliftment in emotions ☐ Improved clarity and acuity of mind ☐ Normalization of thought processes	Abnormal qualities: ☐ Mentally slow, sluggish, spacey ☐ Inability to think quickly or clearly ☐ Hyper, overly rapid thoughts ☐ Inability to focus/hold attention ☐ Hypo traits: Apathy, depression, sadness ☐ Hyper traits: Anxious, obsessive, fearful, angry, short tempered, or irritable, etc.

DIET AND EXERCISE JOURNAL

Date : _____

Diet and Exercise Goals : _____

_____

_____

_____

_____

Meal	List of Food You Ate	Additional Notes
Breakfast		
Lunch		
Dinner		
Snack		

	Exercises	Duration, Repetitions and Additional Notes
Body Balancing Streches		
Core Stability Exercises		
Body Allignment Exercises		

The best way to predict the future is to create it. - Abraham Lincoln

Diet Record Sheet	☐Breakfast ☐Lunch ☐Dinner	
Reactions after a meal	Good	Bad
APPETITE FULLNESS / SATISFACTION SWEET CRAVINGS	Following the meal . . . ☐ Feel full, satisfied ☐ Do NOT have sweet cravings ☐ Do NOT desire more food ☐ Do NOT get hungry soon after ☐ Do NOT need to snack before next meal	Following the meal . . . ☐ Feel physically full, but still hungry ☐ Don't feel satisfied; feel like something was missing from meal ☐ Have desire for sweets ☐ Feel hungry again soon after meal ☐ Need to snack between meals
ENERGY LEVELS	Normal energy response to meal: ☐ Energy is restored after eating ☐ Have good, lasting, "normal" sense of energy and well-being	Poor energy response to meal: ☐ Too much or too little energy ☐ Become hyper, jittery, shaky, nervous, or speedy ☐ Feel hyper, but exhausted "underneath" ☐ Energy drop, fatigue, exhaustion, sleepiness, drowsiness, lethargy, or listlessness
MENTAL EMOTIONAL WELL-BEING	Normal qualities: ☐ Improved well-being ☐ Sense of feeling refueled and restored ☐ Upliftment in emotions ☐ Improved clarity and acuity of mind ☐ Normalization of thought processes	Abnormal qualities: ☐ Mentally slow, sluggish, spacey ☐ Inability to think quickly or clearly ☐ Hyper, overly rapid thoughts ☐ Inability to focus/hold attention ☐ Hypo traits: Apathy, depression, sadness ☐ Hyper traits: Anxious, obsessive, fearful, angry, short tempered, or irritable, etc.

DIET AND EXERCISE JOURNAL

Date : _____

Diet and Exercise Goals : _____

_____

_____

_____

_____

Meal	List of Food You Ate	Additional Notes
Breakfast		
Lunch		
Dinner		
Snack		

	Exercises	Duration, Repetitions and Additional Notes
Body Balancing Streches		
Core Stability Exercises		
Body Allignment Exercises		

In any situation, the best thing you can do is the right thing; the next best thing you can do is the wrong thing; the worst thing you can do is nothing. - Theodore Roosevelt

Diet Record Sheet	☐ Breakfast ☐ Lunch ☐ Dinner	
Reactions after a meal	Good	Bad
APPETITE FULLNESS / SATISFACTION SWEET CRAVINGS	Following the meal . . . ☐ Feel full, satisfied ☐ Do NOT have sweet cravings ☐ Do NOT desire more food ☐ Do NOT get hungry soon after ☐ Do NOT need to snack before next meal	Following the meal . . . ☐ Feel physically full, but still hungry ☐ Don't feel satisfied; feel like something was missing from meal ☐ Have desire for sweets ☐ Feel hungry again soon after meal ☐ Need to snack between meals
ENERGY LEVELS	Normal energy response to meal: ☐ Energy is restored after eating ☐ Have good, lasting, "normal" sense of energy and well-being	Poor energy response to meal: ☐ Too much or too little energy ☐ Become hyper, jittery, shaky, nervous, or speedy ☐ Feel hyper, but exhausted "underneath" ☐ Energy drop, fatigue, exhaustion, sleepiness, drowsiness, lethargy, or listlessness
MENTAL EMOTIONAL WELL-BEING	Normal qualities: ☐ Improved well-being ☐ Sense of feeling refueled and restored ☐ Upliftment in emotions ☐ Improved clarity and acuity of mind ☐ Normalization of thought processes	Abnormal qualities: ☐ Mentally slow, sluggish, spacey ☐ Inability to think quickly or clearly ☐ Hyper, overly rapid thoughts ☐ Inability to focus/hold attention ☐ Hypo traits: Apathy, depression, sadness ☐ Hyper traits: Anxious, obsessive, fearful, angry, short tempered, or irritable, etc.

DIET AND EXERCISE JOURNAL

WEEK 6 / DAY 40

Date : _____

Diet and Exercise Goals : _____

_____

_____

_____

_____

Meal	List of Food You Ate	Additional Notes
Breakfast		
Lunch		
Dinner		
Snack		

	Exercises	Duration, Repetitions and Additional Notes
Body Balancing Streches		
Core Stability Exercises		
Body Allignment Exercises		

Cause change and lead; accept change and survive; resist change and die. - Ray Norda

Diet Record Sheet	☐Breakfast ☐Lunch ☐Dinner	
Reactions after a meal	**Good**	**Bad**
APPETITE FULLNESS / SATISFACTION SWEET CRAVINGS	Following the meal . . . ☐ Feel full, satisfied ☐ Do NOT have sweet cravings ☐ Do NOT desire more food ☐ Do NOT get hungry soon after ☐ Do NOT need to snack before next meal	Following the meal . . . ☐ Feel physically full, but still hungry ☐ Don't feel satisfied; feel like something was missing from meal ☐ Have desire for sweets ☐ Feel hungry again soon after meal ☐ Need to snack between meals
ENERGY LEVELS	Normal energy response to meal: ☐ Energy is restored after eating ☐ Have good, lasting, "normal" sense of energy and well-being	Poor energy response to meal: ☐ Too much or too little energy ☐ Become hyper, jittery, shaky, nervous, or speedy ☐ Feel hyper, but exhausted "underneath" ☐ Energy drop, fatigue, exhaustion, sleepiness, drowsiness, lethargy, or listlessness
MENTAL EMOTIONAL WELL-BEING	Normal qualities: ☐ Improved well-being ☐ Sense of feeling refueled and restored ☐ Upliftment in emotions ☐ Improved clarity and acuity of mind ☐ Normalization of thought processes	Abnormal qualities: ☐ Mentally slow, sluggish, spacey ☐ Inability to think quickly or clearly ☐ Hyper, overly rapid thoughts ☐ Inability to focus/hold attention ☐ Hypo traits: Apathy, depression, sadness ☐ Hyper traits: Anxious, obsessive, fearful, angry, short tempered, or irritable, etc.

DIET AND EXERCISE JOURNAL

Date : _____

Diet and Exercise Goals : _____

_____

_____

_____

_____

Meal	List of Food You Ate	Additional Notes
Breakfast		
Lunch		
Dinner		
Snack		

	Exercises	Duration, Repetitions and Additional Notes
Body Balancing Streches		
Core Stability Exercises		
Body Allignment Exercises		

If you want to make your dreams come true, the first thing you have to do is wake up. - J.M. Power

Diet Record Sheet		☐Breakfast ☐Lunch ☐Dinner
Reactions after a meal	Good	Bad
APPETITE FULLNESS / SATISFACTION SWEET CRAVINGS	Following the meal . . . ☐ Feel full, satisfied ☐ Do NOT have sweet cravings ☐ Do NOT desire more food ☐ Do NOT get hungry soon after ☐ Do NOT need to snack before next meal	Following the meal . . . ☐ Feel physically full, but still hungry ☐ Don't feel satisfied; feel like something was missing from meal ☐ Have desire for sweets ☐ Feel hungry again soon after meal ☐ Need to snack between meals
ENERGY LEVELS	Normal energy response to meal: ☐ Energy is restored after eating ☐ Have good, lasting, "normal" sense of energy and well-being	Poor energy response to meal: ☐ Too much or too little energy ☐ Become hyper, jittery, shaky, nervous, or speedy ☐ Feel hyper, but exhausted "underneath" ☐ Energy drop, fatigue, exhaustion, sleepiness, drowsiness, lethargy, or listlessness
MENTAL EMOTIONAL WELL-BEING	Normal qualities: ☐ Improved well-being ☐ Sense of feeling refueled and restored ☐ Upliftment in emotions ☐ Improved clarity and acuity of mind ☐ Normalization of thought processes	Abnormal qualities: ☐ Mentally slow, sluggish, spacey ☐ Inability to think quickly or clearly ☐ Hyper, overly rapid thoughts ☐ Inability to focus/hold attention ☐ Hypo traits: Apathy, depression, sadness ☐ Hyper traits: Anxious, obsessive, fearful, angry, short tempered, or irritable, etc.

DIET AND EXERCISE JOURNAL   WEEK 6 / DAY 42

Date : _____

Diet and Exercise Goals : _____

_____

_____

_____

_____

Meal	List of Food You Ate	Additional Notes
Breakfast		
Lunch		
Dinner		
Snack		

	Exercises	Duration, Repetitions and Additional Notes
Body Balancing Streches		
Core Stability Exercises		
Body Allignment Exercises		

None of us knows what might happen even the next minute, yet still we go forward. Because we trust.
Because we have Faith. - Paulo Coelho, Brida

Diet Record Sheet		☐Breakfast ☐Lunch ☐Dinner
Reactions after a meal	**Good**	**Bad**
APPETITE FULLNESS / SATISFACTION SWEET CRAVINGS	Following the meal . . . ☐ Feel full, satisfied ☐ Do NOT have sweet cravings ☐ Do NOT desire more food ☐ Do NOT get hungry soon after ☐ Do NOT need to snack before next meal	Following the meal . . . ☐ Feel physically full, but still hungry ☐ Don't feel satisfied; feel like something was missing from meal ☐ Have desire for sweets ☐ Feel hungry again soon after meal ☐ Need to snack between meals
ENERGY LEVELS	Normal energy response to meal: ☐ Energy is restored after eating ☐ Have good, lasting, "normal" sense of energy and well-being	Poor energy response to meal: ☐ Too much or too little energy ☐ Become hyper, jittery, shaky, nervous, or speedy ☐ Feel hyper, but exhausted "underneath" ☐ Energy drop, fatigue, exhaustion, sleepiness, drowsiness, lethargy, or listlessness
MENTAL EMOTIONAL WELL-BEING	Normal qualities: ☐ Improved well-being ☐ Sense of feeling refueled and restored ☐ Upliftment in emotions ☐ Improved clarity and acuity of mind ☐ Normalization of thought processes	Abnormal qualities: ☐ Mentally slow, sluggish, spacey ☐ Inability to think quickly or clearly ☐ Hyper, overly rapid thoughts ☐ Inability to focus/hold attention ☐ Hypo traits: Apathy, depression, sadness ☐ Hyper traits: Anxious, obsessive, fearful, angry, short tempered, or irritable, etc.

DIET AND EXERCISE JOURNAL

WEEK 7 / DAY 43

Date : _____

Diet and Exercise Goals : _____

_____

_____

_____

_____

Meal	List of Food You Ate	Additional Notes
Breakfast		
Lunch		
Dinner		
Snack		

	Exercises	Duration, Repetitions and Additional Notes
Body Balancing Streches		
Core Stability Exercises		
Body Allignment Exercises		

Faith is about doing. You are how you act, not just how you believe. - Mitch Albom

Diet Record Sheet		☐Breakfast ☐Lunch ☐Dinner
Reactions after a meal	Good	Bad
APPETITE FULLNESS / SATISFACTION SWEET CRAVINGS	Following the meal . . . ☐ Feel full, satisfied ☐ Do NOT have sweet cravings ☐ Do NOT desire more food ☐ Do NOT get hungry soon after ☐ Do NOT need to snack before next meal	Following the meal . . . ☐ Feel physically full, but still hungry ☐ Don't feel satisfied; feel like something was missing from meal ☐ Have desire for sweets ☐ Feel hungry again soon after meal ☐ Need to snack between meals
ENERGY LEVELS	Normal energy response to meal: ☐ Energy is restored after eating ☐ Have good, lasting, "normal" sense of energy and well-being	Poor energy response to meal: ☐ Too much or too little energy ☐ Become hyper, jittery, shaky, nervous, or speedy ☐ Feel hyper, but exhausted "underneath" ☐ Energy drop, fatigue, exhaustion, sleepiness, drowsiness, lethargy, or listlessness
MENTAL EMOTIONAL WELL-BEING	Normal qualities: ☐ Improved well-being ☐ Sense of feeling refueled and restored ☐ Upliftment in emotions ☐ Improved clarity and acuity of mind ☐ Normalization of thought processes	Abnormal qualities: ☐ Mentally slow, sluggish, spacey ☐ Inability to think quickly or clearly ☐ Hyper, overly rapid thoughts ☐ Inability to focus/hold attention ☐ Hypo traits: Apathy, depression, sadness ☐ Hyper traits: Anxious, obsessive, fearful, angry, short tempered, or irritable, etc.

DIET AND EXERCISE JOURNAL

WEEK 7 / DAY 44

Date : _____

Diet and Exercise Goals : _____

_____

_____

_____

_____

Meal	List of Food You Ate	Additional Notes
Breakfast		
Lunch		
Dinner		
Snack		

	Exercises	Duration, Repetitions and Additional Notes
Body Balancing Streches		
Core Stability Exercises		
Body Allignment Exercises		

Yesterday is gone. Tomorrow has not yet come. We have only today. Let us begin. - Mother Teresa

Diet Record Sheet		☐Breakfast ☐Lunch ☐Dinner
Reactions after a meal	**Good**	**Bad**
APPETITE FULLNESS / SATISFACTION SWEET CRAVINGS	Following the meal . . . ☐ Feel full, satisfied ☐ Do NOT have sweet cravings ☐ Do NOT desire more food ☐ Do NOT get hungry soon after ☐ Do NOT need to snack before next meal	Following the meal . . . ☐ Feel physically full, but still hungry ☐ Don't feel satisfied; feel like something was missing from meal ☐ Have desire for sweets ☐ Feel hungry again soon after meal ☐ Need to snack between meals
ENERGY LEVELS	Normal energy response to meal: ☐ Energy is restored after eating ☐ Have good, lasting, "normal" sense of energy and well-being	Poor energy response to meal: ☐ Too much or too little energy ☐ Become hyper, jittery, shaky, nervous, or speedy ☐ Feel hyper, but exhausted "underneath" ☐ Energy drop, fatigue, exhaustion, sleepiness, drowsiness, lethargy, or listlessness
MENTAL EMOTIONAL WELL-BEING	Normal qualities: ☐ Improved well-being ☐ Sense of feeling refueled and restored ☐ Upliftment in emotions ☐ Improved clarity and acuity of mind ☐ Normalization of thought processes	Abnormal qualities: ☐ Mentally slow, sluggish, spacey ☐ Inability to think quickly or clearly ☐ Hyper, overly rapid thoughts ☐ Inability to focus/hold attention ☐ Hypo traits: Apathy, depression, sadness ☐ Hyper traits: Anxious, obsessive, fearful, angry, short tempered, or irritable, etc.

DIET AND EXERCISE JOURNAL   WEEK 7 / DAY 45

Date : _____

Diet and Exercise Goals : _____

_____

_____

_____

_____

Meal	List of Food You Ate	Additional Notes
Breakfast		
Lunch		
Dinner		
Snack		

	Exercises	Duration, Repetitions and Additional Notes
Body Balancing Streches		
Core Stability Exercises		
Body Allignment Exercises		

You may delay, but time will not. - Benjamin Franklin

Diet Record Sheet	☐Breakfast ☐Lunch ☐Dinner	
Reactions after a meal	**Good**	**Bad**
APPETITE FULLNESS / SATISFACTION SWEET CRAVINGS	Following the meal . . . ☐ Feel full, satisfied ☐ Do NOT have sweet cravings ☐ Do NOT desire more food ☐ Do NOT get hungry soon after ☐ Do NOT need to snack before next meal	Following the meal . . . ☐ Feel physically full, but still hungry ☐ Don't feel satisfied; feel like something was missing from meal ☐ Have desire for sweets ☐ Feel hungry again soon after meal ☐ Need to snack between meals
ENERGY LEVELS	Normal energy response to meal: ☐ Energy is restored after eating ☐ Have good, lasting, "normal" sense of energy and well-being	Poor energy response to meal: ☐ Too much or too little energy ☐ Become hyper, jittery, shaky, nervous, or speedy ☐ Feel hyper, but exhausted "underneath" ☐ Energy drop, fatigue, exhaustion, sleepiness, drowsiness, lethargy, or listlessness
MENTAL EMOTIONAL WELL-BEING	Normal qualities: ☐ Improved well-being ☐ Sense of feeling refueled and restored ☐ Upliftment in emotions ☐ Improved clarity and acuity of mind ☐ Normalization of thought processes	Abnormal qualities: ☐ Mentally slow, sluggish, spacey ☐ Inability to think quickly or clearly ☐ Hyper, overly rapid thoughts ☐ Inability to focus/hold attention ☐ Hypo traits: Apathy, depression, sadness ☐ Hyper traits: Anxious, obsessive, fearful, angry, short tempered, or irritable, etc.

DIET AND EXERCISE JOURNAL

Date : _____

Diet and Exercise Goals : _____

_____

_____

_____

_____

Meal	List of Food You Ate	Additional Notes
Breakfast		
Lunch		
Dinner		
Snack		

	Exercises	Duration, Repetitions and Additional Notes
Body Balancing Streches		
Core Stability Exercises		
Body Allignment Exercises		

Breathe. Let go. And remind yourself that this very moment is the only one you know
you have for sure. - Oprah Winfrey

Diet Record Sheet	☐Breakfast ☐Lunch ☐Dinner

Reactions after a meal	Good	Bad
APPETITE FULLNESS / SATISFACTION SWEET CRAVINGS	Following the meal . . . ☐ Feel full, satisfied ☐ Do NOT have sweet cravings ☐ Do NOT desire more food ☐ Do NOT get hungry soon after ☐ Do NOT need to snack before next meal	Following the meal . . . ☐ Feel physically full, but still hungry ☐ Don't feel satisfied; feel like something was missing from meal ☐ Have desire for sweets ☐ Feel hungry again soon after meal ☐ Need to snack between meals
ENERGY LEVELS	Normal energy response to meal: ☐ Energy is restored after eating ☐ Have good, lasting, "normal" sense of energy and well-being	Poor energy response to meal: ☐ Too much or too little energy ☐ Become hyper, jittery, shaky, nervous, or speedy ☐ Feel hyper, but exhausted "underneath" ☐ Energy drop, fatigue, exhaustion, sleepiness, drowsiness, lethargy, or listlessness
MENTAL EMOTIONAL WELL-BEING	Normal qualities: ☐ Improved well-being ☐ Sense of feeling refueled and restored ☐ Upliftment in emotions ☐ Improved clarity and acuity of mind ☐ Normalization of thought processes	Abnormal qualities: ☐ Mentally slow, sluggish, spacey ☐ Inability to think quickly or clearly ☐ Hyper, overly rapid thoughts ☐ Inability to focus/hold attention ☐ Hypo traits: Apathy, depression, sadness ☐ Hyper traits: Anxious, obsessive, fearful, angry, short tempered, or irritable, etc.

DIET AND EXERCISE JOURNAL

WEEK 7 / DAY 47

Date : _____

Diet and Exercise Goals : _____

_____

_____

_____

_____

Meal	List of Food You Ate	Additional Notes
Breakfast		
Lunch		
Dinner		
Snack		

	Exercises	Duration, Repetitions and Additional Notes
Body Balancing Streches		
Core Stability Exercises		
Body Allignment Exercises		

If you want your life to change, your choices must change,
today is the best day of your life to begin. - rewirethoughts.com

Diet Record Sheet		☐Breakfast ☐Lunch ☐Dinner
Reactions after a meal	**Good**	**Bad**
APPETITE FULLNESS / SATISFACTION SWEET CRAVINGS	Following the meal . . . ☐ Feel full, satisfied ☐ Do NOT have sweet cravings ☐ Do NOT desire more food ☐ Do NOT get hungry soon after ☐ Do NOT need to snack before next meal	Following the meal . . . ☐ Feel physically full, but still hungry ☐ Don't feel satisfied; feel like something was missing from meal ☐ Have desire for sweets ☐ Feel hungry again soon after meal ☐ Need to snack between meals
ENERGY LEVELS	Normal energy response to meal: ☐ Energy is restored after eating ☐ Have good, lasting, "normal" sense of energy and well-being	Poor energy response to meal: ☐ Too much or too little energy ☐ Become hyper, jittery, shaky, nervous, or speedy ☐ Feel hyper, but exhausted "underneath" ☐ Energy drop, fatigue, exhaustion, sleepiness, drowsiness, lethargy, or listlessness
MENTAL EMOTIONAL WELL-BEING	Normal qualities: ☐ Improved well-being ☐ Sense of feeling refueled and restored ☐ Upliftment in emotions ☐ Improved clarity and acuity of mind ☐ Normalization of thought processes	Abnormal qualities: ☐ Mentally slow, sluggish, spacey ☐ Inability to think quickly or clearly ☐ Hyper, overly rapid thoughts ☐ Inability to focus/hold attention ☐ Hypo traits: Apathy, depression, sadness ☐ Hyper traits: Anxious, obsessive, fearful, angry, short tempered, or irritable, etc.

DIET AND EXERCISE JOURNAL   WEEK 7 / DAY 48

Date : _____

Diet and Exercise Goals : _____

_____

_____

_____

_____

Meal	List of Food You Ate	Additional Notes
Breakfast		
Lunch		
Dinner		
Snack		

	Exercises	Duration, Repetitions and Additional Notes
Body Balancing Streches		
Core Stability Exercises		
Body Allignment Exercises		

The best six doctors anywhere and no one can deny it are sunshine,
water, rest, air, exercise and diet. - Wayne Fields

Diet Record Sheet	☐Breakfast ☐Lunch ☐Dinner	
Reactions after a meal	**Good**	**Bad**
APPETITE FULLNESS / SATISFACTION SWEET CRAVINGS	Following the meal . . . ☐ Feel full, satisfied ☐ Do NOT have sweet cravings ☐ Do NOT desire more food ☐ Do NOT get hungry soon after ☐ Do NOT need to snack before next meal	Following the meal . . . ☐ Feel physically full, but still hungry ☐ Don't feel satisfied; feel like something was missing from meal ☐ Have desire for sweets ☐ Feel hungry again soon after meal ☐ Need to snack between meals
ENERGY LEVELS	Normal energy response to meal: ☐ Energy is restored after eating ☐ Have good, lasting, "normal" sense of energy and well-being	Poor energy response to meal: ☐ Too much or too little energy ☐ Become hyper, jittery, shaky, nervous, or speedy ☐ Feel hyper, but exhausted "underneath" ☐ Energy drop, fatigue, exhaustion, sleepiness, drowsiness, lethargy, or listlessness
MENTAL EMOTIONAL WELL-BEING	Normal qualities: ☐ Improved well-being ☐ Sense of feeling refueled and restored ☐ Upliftment in emotions ☐ Improved clarity and acuity of mind ☐ Normalization of thought processes	Abnormal qualities: ☐ Mentally slow, sluggish, spacey ☐ Inability to think quickly or clearly ☐ Hyper, overly rapid thoughts ☐ Inability to focus/hold attention ☐ Hypo traits: Apathy, depression, sadness ☐ Hyper traits: Anxious, obsessive, fearful, angry, short tempered, or irritable, etc.

DIET AND EXERCISE JOURNAL

WEEK 7 / DAY 49

Date : _____

Diet and Exercise Goals : _____

_____

_____

_____

_____

_____

Meal	List of Food You Ate	Additional Notes
Breakfast		
Lunch		
Dinner		
Snack		

	Exercises	Duration, Repetitions and Additional Notes
Body Balancing Streches		
Core Stability Exercises		
Body Allignment Exercises		

You don't always get what wish for, you get what you work for! - Author Unknown

Diet Record Sheet		☐Breakfast ☐Lunch ☐Dinner
Reactions after a meal	**Good**	**Bad**
APPETITE FULLNESS / SATISFACTION SWEET CRAVINGS	Following the meal . . . ☐ Feel full, satisfied ☐ Do NOT have sweet cravings ☐ Do NOT desire more food ☐ Do NOT get hungry soon after ☐ Do NOT need to snack before next meal	Following the meal . . . ☐ Feel physically full, but still hungry ☐ Don't feel satisfied; feel like something was missing from meal ☐ Have desire for sweets ☐ Feel hungry again soon after meal ☐ Need to snack between meals
ENERGY LEVELS	Normal energy response to meal: ☐ Energy is restored after eating ☐ Have good, lasting, "normal" sense of energy and well-being	Poor energy response to meal: ☐ Too much or too little energy ☐ Become hyper, jittery, shaky, nervous, or speedy ☐ Feel hyper, but exhausted "underneath" ☐ Energy drop, fatigue, exhaustion, sleepiness, drowsiness, lethargy, or listlessness
MENTAL EMOTIONAL WELL-BEING	Normal qualities: ☐ Improved well-being ☐ Sense of feeling refueled and restored ☐ Upliftment in emotions ☐ Improved clarity and acuity of mind ☐ Normalization of thought processes	Abnormal qualities: ☐ Mentally slow, sluggish, spacey ☐ Inability to think quickly or clearly ☐ Hyper, overly rapid thoughts ☐ Inability to focus/hold attention ☐ Hypo traits: Apathy, depression, sadness ☐ Hyper traits: Anxious, obsessive, fearful, angry, short tempered, or irritable, etc.

Week 8: Scoliosis Symptoms Review

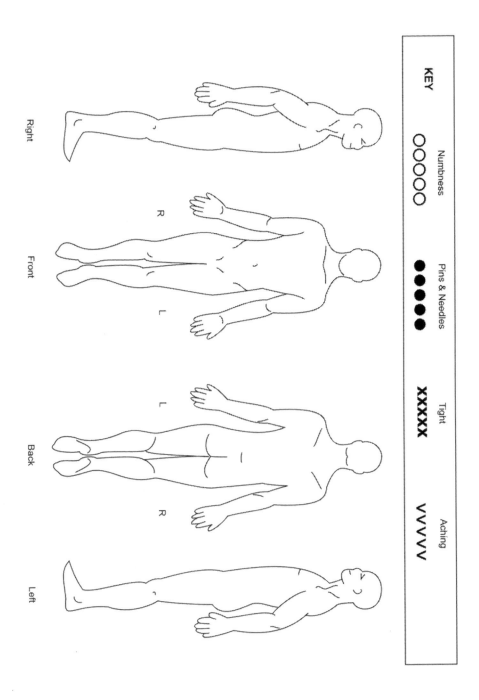

Week 8: Trigger Point Mapping

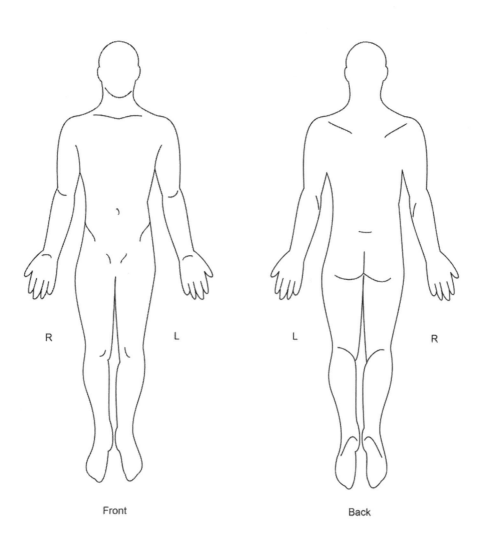

R   L   L   R

Front   Back

DIET AND EXERCISE JOURNAL   WEEK 8 / DAY 50

Date : _____

Diet and Exercise Goals : _____

_____

_____

_____

_____

Meal	List of Food You Ate	Additional Notes
Breakfast		
Lunch		
Dinner		
Snack		

	Exercises	Duration, Repetitions and Additional Notes
Body Balancing Streches		
Core Stability Exercises		
Body Allignment Exercises		

Don't start your day with the broken pieces of yesterday. Don't overstay in the past and waste time for your future. Don't spend your time looking at what you left behind because you'll miss what's waiting for you ahead. - Author Unknown

Diet Record Sheet	☐Breakfast ☐Lunch ☐Dinner	
Reactions after a meal	Good	Bad
APPETITE FULLNESS / SATISFACTION SWEET CRAVINGS	Following the meal . . . ☐ Feel full, satisfied ☐ Do NOT have sweet cravings ☐ Do NOT desire more food ☐ Do NOT get hungry soon after ☐ Do NOT need to snack before next meal	Following the meal . . . ☐ Feel physically full, but still hungry ☐ Don't feel satisfied; feel like something was missing from meal ☐ Have desire for sweets ☐ Feel hungry again soon after meal ☐ Need to snack between meals
ENERGY LEVELS	Normal energy response to meal: ☐ Energy is restored after eating ☐ Have good, lasting, "normal" sense of energy and well-being	Poor energy response to meal: ☐ Too much or too little energy ☐ Become hyper, jittery, shaky, nervous, or speedy ☐ Feel hyper, but exhausted "underneath" ☐ Energy drop, fatigue, exhaustion, sleepiness, drowsiness, lethargy, or listlessness
MENTAL EMOTIONAL WELL-BEING	Normal qualities: ☐ Improved well-being ☐ Sense of feeling refueled and restored ☐ Upliftment in emotions ☐ Improved clarity and acuity of mind ☐ Normalization of thought processes	Abnormal qualities: ☐ Mentally slow, sluggish, spacey ☐ Inability to think quickly or clearly ☐ Hyper, overly rapid thoughts ☐ Inability to focus/hold attention ☐ Hypo traits: Apathy, depression, sadness ☐ Hyper traits: Anxious, obsessive, fearful, angry, short tempered, or irritable, etc.

DIET AND EXERCISE JOURNAL   WEEK 8 / DAY 51

Date : _____

Diet and Exercise Goals : _____

_____

_____

_____

_____

Meal	List of Food You Ate	Additional Notes
Breakfast		
Lunch		
Dinner		
Snack		

	Exercises	Duration, Repetitions and Additional Notes
Body Balancing Streches		
Core Stability Exercises		
Body Allignment Exercises		

Clear your mind of can't. - Samuel Johnson

Diet Record Sheet	☐Breakfast ☐Lunch ☐Dinner	
Reactions after a meal	Good	Bad
APPETITE FULLNESS / SATISFACTION SWEET CRAVINGS	Following the meal . . . ☐ Feel full, satisfied ☐ Do NOT have sweet cravings ☐ Do NOT desire more food ☐ Do NOT get hungry soon after ☐ Do NOT need to snack before next meal	Following the meal . . . ☐ Feel physically full, but still hungry ☐ Don't feel satisfied; feel like something was missing from meal ☐ Have desire for sweets ☐ Feel hungry again soon after meal ☐ Need to snack between meals
ENERGY LEVELS	Normal energy response to meal: ☐ Energy is restored after eating ☐ Have good, lasting, "normal" sense of energy and well-being	Poor energy response to meal: ☐ Too much or too little energy ☐ Become hyper, jittery, shaky, nervous, or speedy ☐ Feel hyper, but exhausted "underneath" ☐ Energy drop, fatigue, exhaustion, sleepiness, drowsiness, lethargy, or listlessness
MENTAL EMOTIONAL WELL-BEING	Normal qualities: ☐ Improved well-being ☐ Sense of feeling refueled and restored ☐ Upliftment in emotions ☐ Improved clarity and acuity of mind ☐ Normalization of thought processes	Abnormal qualities: ☐ Mentally slow, sluggish, spacey ☐ Inability to think quickly or clearly ☐ Hyper, overly rapid thoughts ☐ Inability to focus/hold attention ☐ Hypo traits: Apathy, depression, sadness ☐ Hyper traits: Anxious, obsessive, fearful, angry, short tempered, or irritable, etc.

DIET AND EXERCISE JOURNAL

WEEK 8 / DAY 52

Date : _____

Diet and Exercise Goals : _____

_____

_____

_____

_____

Meal	List of Food You Ate	Additional Notes
Breakfast		
Lunch		
Dinner		
Snack		

	Exercises	Duration, Repetitions and Additional Notes
Body Balancing Streches		
Core Stability Exercises		
Body Allignment Exercises		

The only bad workout is the one that didn't happen. - Author Unknown

Diet Record Sheet	□Breakfast □Lunch □Dinner	
Reactions after a meal	**Good**	**Bad**
APPETITE FULLNESS / SATISFACTION SWEET CRAVINGS	Following the meal . . . ☐ Feel full, satisfied ☐ Do NOT have sweet cravings ☐ Do NOT desire more food ☐ Do NOT get hungry soon after ☐ Do NOT need to snack before next meal	Following the meal . . . ☐ Feel physically full, but still hungry ☐ Don't feel satisfied; feel like something was missing from meal ☐ Have desire for sweets ☐ Feel hungry again soon after meal ☐ Need to snack between meals
ENERGY LEVELS	Normal energy response to meal: ☐ Energy is restored after eating ☐ Have good, lasting, "normal" sense of energy and well-being	Poor energy response to meal: ☐ Too much or too little energy ☐ Become hyper, jittery, shaky, nervous, or speedy ☐ Feel hyper, but exhausted "underneath" ☐ Energy drop, fatigue, exhaustion, sleepiness, drowsiness, lethargy, or listlessness
MENTAL EMOTIONAL WELL-BEING	Normal qualities: ☐ Improved well-being ☐ Sense of feeling refueled and restored ☐ Upliftment in emotions ☐ Improved clarity and acuity of mind ☐ Normalization of thought processes	Abnormal qualities: ☐ Mentally slow, sluggish, spacey ☐ Inability to think quickly or clearly ☐ Hyper, overly rapid thoughts ☐ Inability to focus/hold attention ☐ Hypo traits: Apathy, depression, sadness ☐ Hyper traits: Anxious, obsessive, fearful, angry, short tempered, or irritable, etc.

DIET AND EXERCISE JOURNAL　　　　WEEK 8 / DAY 53

Date :　_____

Diet and Exercise Goals :　_____

_____

_____

_____

_____

Meal	List of Food You Ate	Additional Notes
Breakfast		
Lunch		
Dinner		
Snack		

	Exercises	Duration, Repetitions and Additional Notes
Body Balancing Streches		
Core Stability Exercises		
Body Allignment Exercises		

It's never a question of can you, but will you? - Author Unknown

Diet Record Sheet	☐Breakfast ☐Lunch ☐Dinner	
Reactions after a meal	Good	Bad
APPETITE FULLNESS / SATISFACTION SWEET CRAVINGS	Following the meal . . . ☐ Feel full, satisfied ☐ Do NOT have sweet cravings ☐ Do NOT desire more food ☐ Do NOT get hungry soon after ☐ Do NOT need to snack before next meal	Following the meal . . . ☐ Feel physically full, but still hungry ☐ Don't feel satisfied; feel like something was missing from meal ☐ Have desire for sweets ☐ Feel hungry again soon after meal ☐ Need to snack between meals
ENERGY LEVELS	Normal energy response to meal: ☐ Energy is restored after eating ☐ Have good, lasting, "normal" sense of energy and well-being	Poor energy response to meal: ☐ Too much or too little energy ☐ Become hyper, jittery, shaky, nervous, or speedy ☐ Feel hyper, but exhausted "underneath" ☐ Energy drop, fatigue, exhaustion, sleepiness, drowsiness, lethargy, or listlessness
MENTAL EMOTIONAL WELL-BEING	Normal qualities: ☐ Improved well-being ☐ Sense of feeling refueled and restored ☐ Upliftment in emotions ☐ Improved clarity and acuity of mind ☐ Normalization of thought processes	Abnormal qualities: ☐ Mentally slow, sluggish, spacey ☐ Inability to think quickly or clearly ☐ Hyper, overly rapid thoughts ☐ Inability to focus/hold attention ☐ Hypo traits: Apathy, depression, sadness ☐ Hyper traits: Anxious, obsessive, fearful, angry, short tempered, or irritable, etc.

DIET AND EXERCISE JOURNAL   WEEK 8 / DAY 54

Date : _____

Diet and Exercise Goals : _____

_____

_____

_____

_____

Meal	List of Food You Ate	Additional Notes
Breakfast		
Lunch		
Dinner		
Snack		

	Exercises	Duration, Repetitions and Additional Notes
Body Balancing Streches		
Core Stability Exercises		
Body Allignment Exercises		

If you talk to your friend the way you talk to your body, you'd have no friends left. - Author Unknown

Diet Record Sheet	☐Breakfast ☐Lunch ☐Dinner	
Reactions after a meal	**Good**	**Bad**
APPETITE FULLNESS / SATISFACTION SWEET CRAVINGS	Following the meal . . . ☐ Feel full, satisfied ☐ Do NOT have sweet cravings ☐ Do NOT desire more food ☐ Do NOT get hungry soon after ☐ Do NOT need to snack before next meal	Following the meal . . . ☐ Feel physically full, but still hungry ☐ Don't feel satisfied; feel like something was missing from meal ☐ Have desire for sweets ☐ Feel hungry again soon after meal ☐ Need to snack between meals
ENERGY LEVELS	Normal energy response to meal: ☐ Energy is restored after eating ☐ Have good, lasting, "normal" sense of energy and well-being	Poor energy response to meal: ☐ Too much or too little energy ☐ Become hyper, jittery, shaky, nervous, or speedy ☐ Feel hyper, but exhausted "underneath" ☐ Energy drop, fatigue, exhaustion, sleepiness, drowsiness, lethargy, or listlessness
MENTAL EMOTIONAL WELL-BEING	Normal qualities: ☐ Improved well-being ☐ Sense of feeling refueled and restored ☐ Upliftment in emotions ☐ Improved clarity and acuity of mind ☐ Normalization of thought processes	Abnormal qualities: ☐ Mentally slow, sluggish, spacey ☐ Inability to think quickly or clearly ☐ Hyper, overly rapid thoughts ☐ Inability to focus/hold attention ☐ Hypo traits: Apathy, depression, sadness ☐ Hyper traits: Anxious, obsessive, fearful, angry, short tempered, or irritable, etc.

DIET AND EXERCISE JOURNAL   WEEK 8 / DAY 55

Date : _____

Diet and Exercise Goals : _____

_____

_____

_____

_____

Meal	List of Food You Ate	Additional Notes
Breakfast		
Lunch		
Dinner		
Snack		

	Exercises	Duration, Repetitions and Additional Notes
Body Balancing Streches		
Core Stability Exercises		
Body Allignment Exercises		

Diets, like clothes, should be tailored to you. - Joan Rivers

Diet Record Sheet	☐ Breakfast ☐ Lunch ☐ Dinner	
Reactions after a meal	**Good**	**Bad**
APPETITE FULLNESS / SATISFACTION SWEET CRAVINGS	Following the meal . . . ☐ Feel full, satisfied ☐ Do NOT have sweet cravings ☐ Do NOT desire more food ☐ Do NOT get hungry soon after ☐ Do NOT need to snack before next meal	Following the meal . . . ☐ Feel physically full, but still hungry ☐ Don't feel satisfied; feel like something was missing from meal ☐ Have desire for sweets ☐ Feel hungry again soon after meal ☐ Need to snack between meals
ENERGY LEVELS	Normal energy response to meal: ☐ Energy is restored after eating ☐ Have good, lasting, "normal" sense of energy and well-being	Poor energy response to meal: ☐ Too much or too little energy ☐ Become hyper, jittery, shaky, nervous, or speedy ☐ Feel hyper, but exhausted "underneath" ☐ Energy drop, fatigue, exhaustion, sleepiness, drowsiness, lethargy, or listlessness
MENTAL EMOTIONAL WELL-BEING	Normal qualities: ☐ Improved well-being ☐ Sense of feeling refueled and restored ☐ Upliftment in emotions ☐ Improved clarity and acuity of mind ☐ Normalization of thought processes	Abnormal qualities: ☐ Mentally slow, sluggish, spacey ☐ Inability to think quickly or clearly ☐ Hyper, overly rapid thoughts ☐ Inability to focus/hold attention ☐ Hypo traits: Apathy, depression, sadness ☐ Hyper traits: Anxious, obsessive, fearful, angry, short tempered, or irritable, etc.

DIET AND EXERCISE JOURNAL   WEEK 8 / DAY 56

Date : _____

Diet and Exercise Goals : _____

_____

_____

_____

_____

Meal	List of Food You Ate	Additional Notes
Breakfast		
Lunch		
Dinner		
Snack		

	Exercises	Duration, Repetitions and Additional Notes
Body Balancing Streches		
Core Stability Exercises		
Body Allignment Exercises		

The wish for healing has always been half of health. - Lucius Annaeus Seneca

Diet Record Sheet	☐Breakfast ☐Lunch ☐Dinner	
Reactions after a meal	**Good**	**Bad**
APPETITE FULLNESS / SATISFACTION SWEET CRAVINGS	Following the meal . . . ☐ Feel full, satisfied ☐ Do NOT have sweet cravings ☐ Do NOT desire more food ☐ Do NOT get hungry soon after ☐ Do NOT need to snack before next meal	Following the meal . . . ☐ Feel physically full, but still hungry ☐ Don't feel satisfied; feel like something was missing from meal ☐ Have desire for sweets ☐ Feel hungry again soon after meal ☐ Need to snack between meals
ENERGY LEVELS	Normal energy response to meal: ☐ Energy is restored after eating ☐ Have good, lasting, "normal" sense of energy and well-being	Poor energy response to meal: ☐ Too much or too little energy ☐ Become hyper, jittery, shaky, nervous, or speedy ☐ Feel hyper, but exhausted "underneath" ☐ Energy drop, fatigue, exhaustion, sleepiness, drowsiness, lethargy, or listlessness
MENTAL EMOTIONAL WELL-BEING	Normal qualities: ☐ Improved well-being ☐ Sense of feeling refueled and restored ☐ Upliftment in emotions ☐ Improved clarity and acuity of mind ☐ Normalization of thought processes	Abnormal qualities: ☐ Mentally slow, sluggish, spacey ☐ Inability to think quickly or clearly ☐ Hyper, overly rapid thoughts ☐ Inability to focus/hold attention ☐ Hypo traits: Apathy, depression, sadness ☐ Hyper traits: Anxious, obsessive, fearful, angry, short tempered, or irritable, etc.

DIET AND EXERCISE JOURNAL   WEEK 9 / DAY 57

Date : _____

Diet and Exercise Goals : _____

_____

_____

_____

_____

Meal	List of Food You Ate	Additional Notes
Breakfast		
Lunch		
Dinner		
Snack		

	Exercises	Duration, Repetitions and Additional Notes
Body Balancing Streches		
Core Stability Exercises		
Body Allignment Exercises		

Nothing in life is to be feared, it is only to be understood. Now is the time to understand more,
so that we may fear less. - Marie Curie

Diet Record Sheet	☐Breakfast	☐Lunch	☐Dinner
Reactions after a meal	**Good**		**Bad**
APPETITE FULLNESS / SATISFACTION SWEET CRAVINGS	Following the meal . . . ☐ Feel full, satisfied ☐ Do NOT have sweet cravings ☐ Do NOT desire more food ☐ Do NOT get hungry soon after ☐ Do NOT need to snack before next meal		Following the meal . . . ☐ Feel physically full, but still hungry ☐ Don't feel satisfied; feel like something was missing from meal ☐ Have desire for sweets ☐ Feel hungry again soon after meal ☐ Need to snack between meals
ENERGY LEVELS	Normal energy response to meal: ☐ Energy is restored after eating ☐ Have good, lasting, "normal" sense of energy and well-being		Poor energy response to meal: ☐ Too much or too little energy ☐ Become hyper, jittery, shaky, nervous, or speedy ☐ Feel hyper, but exhausted "underneath" ☐ Energy drop, fatigue, exhaustion, sleepiness, drowsiness, lethargy, or listlessness
MENTAL EMOTIONAL WELL-BEING	Normal qualities: ☐ Improved well-being ☐ Sense of feeling refueled and restored ☐ Upliftment in emotions ☐ Improved clarity and acuity of mind ☐ Normalization of thought processes		Abnormal qualities: ☐ Mentally slow, sluggish, spacey ☐ Inability to think quickly or clearly ☐ Hyper, overly rapid thoughts ☐ Inability to focus/hold attention ☐ Hypo traits: Apathy, depression, sadness ☐ Hyper traits: Anxious, obsessive, fearful, angry, short tempered, or irritable, etc.

DIET AND EXERCISE JOURNAL

WEEK 9 / DAY 58

Date : _____

Diet and Exercise Goals : _____

_____

_____

_____

_____

Meal	List of Food You Ate	Additional Notes
Breakfast		
Lunch		
Dinner		
Snack		

	Exercises	Duration, Repetitions and Additional Notes
Body Balancing Streches		
Core Stability Exercises		
Body Allignment Exercises		

Attitude is a little thing that makes a big difference. - Winston Churchill

Diet Record Sheet	☐Breakfast ☐Lunch ☐Dinner	
Reactions after a meal	Good	Bad
APPETITE FULLNESS / SATISFACTION SWEET CRAVINGS	Following the meal . . . ☐ Feel full, satisfied ☐ Do NOT have sweet cravings ☐ Do NOT desire more food ☐ Do NOT get hungry soon after ☐ Do NOT need to snack before next meal	Following the meal . . . ☐ Feel physically full, but still hungry ☐ Don't feel satisfied; feel like something was missing from meal ☐ Have desire for sweets ☐ Feel hungry again soon after meal ☐ Need to snack between meals
ENERGY LEVELS	Normal energy response to meal: ☐ Energy is restored after eating ☐ Have good, lasting, "normal" sense of energy and well-being	Poor energy response to meal: ☐ Too much or too little energy ☐ Become hyper, jittery, shaky, nervous, or speedy ☐ Feel hyper, but exhausted "underneath" ☐ Energy drop, fatigue, exhaustion, sleepiness, drowsiness, lethargy, or listlessness
MENTAL EMOTIONAL WELL-BEING	Normal qualities: ☐ Improved well-being ☐ Sense of feeling refueled and restored ☐ Upliftment in emotions ☐ Improved clarity and acuity of mind ☐ Normalization of thought processes	Abnormal qualities: ☐ Mentally slow, sluggish, spacey ☐ Inability to think quickly or clearly ☐ Hyper, overly rapid thoughts ☐ Inability to focus/hold attention ☐ Hypo traits: Apathy, depression, sadness ☐ Hyper traits: Anxious, obsessive, fearful, angry, short tempered, or irritable, etc.

DIET AND EXERCISE JOURNAL

Date : _____

Diet and Exercise Goals : _____

_____

_____

_____

_____

Meal	List of Food You Ate	Additional Notes
Breakfast		
Lunch		
Dinner		
Snack		

	Exercises	Duration, Repetitions and Additional Notes
Body Balancing Streches		
Core Stability Exercises		
Body Allignment Exercises		

The future belongs to those who see possibilities before they become obvious. - John Scully

Diet Record Sheet	☐Breakfast ☐Lunch ☐Dinner	
Reactions after a meal	**Good**	**Bad**
APPETITE FULLNESS / SATISFACTION SWEET CRAVINGS	Following the meal . . . ☐ Feel full, satisfied ☐ Do NOT have sweet cravings ☐ Do NOT desire more food ☐ Do NOT get hungry soon after ☐ Do NOT need to snack before next meal	Following the meal . . . ☐ Feel physically full, but still hungry ☐ Don't feel satisfied; feel like something was missing from meal ☐ Have desire for sweets ☐ Feel hungry again soon after meal ☐ Need to snack between meals
ENERGY LEVELS	Normal energy response to meal: ☐ Energy is restored after eating ☐ Have good, lasting, "normal" sense of energy and well-being	Poor energy response to meal: ☐ Too much or too little energy ☐ Become hyper, jittery, shaky, nervous, or speedy ☐ Feel hyper, but exhausted "underneath" ☐ Energy drop, fatigue, exhaustion, sleepiness, drowsiness, lethargy, or listlessness
MENTAL EMOTIONAL WELL-BEING	Normal qualities: ☐ Improved well-being ☐ Sense of feeling refueled and restored ☐ Upliftment in emotions ☐ Improved clarity and acuity of mind ☐ Normalization of thought processes	Abnormal qualities: ☐ Mentally slow, sluggish, spacey ☐ Inability to think quickly or clearly ☐ Hyper, overly rapid thoughts ☐ Inability to focus/hold attention ☐ Hypo traits: Apathy, depression, sadness ☐ Hyper traits: Anxious, obsessive, fearful, angry, short tempered, or irritable, etc.

DIET AND EXERCISE JOURNAL

WEEK 9 / DAY 60

Date : _____

Diet and Exercise Goals : _____

_____

_____

_____

_____

Meal	List of Food You Ate	Additional Notes
Breakfast		
Lunch		
Dinner		
Snack		

	Exercises	Duration, Repetitions and Additional Notes
Body Balancing Streches		
Core Stability Exercises		
Body Allignment Exercises		

Mastering others is strength. Mastering yourself is true power. - Lao Tzu

Diet Record Sheet	☐Breakfast ☐Lunch ☐Dinner	
Reactions after a meal	**Good**	**Bad**
APPETITE FULLNESS / SATISFACTION SWEET CRAVINGS	Following the meal . . . ☐ Feel full, satisfied ☐ Do NOT have sweet cravings ☐ Do NOT desire more food ☐ Do NOT get hungry soon after ☐ Do NOT need to snack before next meal	Following the meal . . . ☐ Feel physically full, but still hungry ☐ Don't feel satisfied; feel like something was missing from meal ☐ Have desire for sweets ☐ Feel hungry again soon after meal ☐ Need to snack between meals
ENERGY LEVELS	Normal energy response to meal: ☐ Energy is restored after eating ☐ Have good, lasting, "normal" sense of energy and well-being	Poor energy response to meal: ☐ Too much or too little energy ☐ Become hyper, jittery, shaky, nervous, or speedy ☐ Feel hyper, but exhausted "underneath" ☐ Energy drop, fatigue, exhaustion, sleepiness, drowsiness, lethargy, or listlessness
MENTAL EMOTIONAL WELL-BEING	Normal qualities: ☐ Improved well-being ☐ Sense of feeling refueled and restored ☐ Upliftment in emotions ☐ Improved clarity and acuity of mind ☐ Normalization of thought processes	Abnormal qualities: ☐ Mentally slow, sluggish, spacey ☐ Inability to think quickly or clearly ☐ Hyper, overly rapid thoughts ☐ Inability to focus/hold attention ☐ Hypo traits: Apathy, depression, sadness ☐ Hyper traits: Anxious, obsessive, fearful, angry, short tempered, or irritable, etc.

DIET AND EXERCISE JOURNAL

WEEK 9 / DAY 61

Date : _____

Diet and Exercise Goals : _____

_____

_____

_____

_____

Meal	List of Food You Ate	Additional Notes
Breakfast		
Lunch		
Dinner		
Snack		

	Exercises	Duration, Repetitions and Additional Notes
Body Balancing Streches		
Core Stability Exercises		
Body Allignment Exercises		

We are all here for some special reason. Stop being a prisoner of your past.
Become the architect of your future. - Robin Sharma

Diet Record Sheet	☐Breakfast ☐Lunch ☐Dinner	
Reactions after a meal	Good	Bad
APPETITE FULLNESS / SATISFACTION SWEET CRAVINGS	Following the meal . . . ☐ Feel full, satisfied ☐ Do NOT have sweet cravings ☐ Do NOT desire more food ☐ Do NOT get hungry soon after ☐ Do NOT need to snack before next meal	Following the meal . . . ☐ Feel physically full, but still hungry ☐ Don't feel satisfied; feel like something was missing from meal ☐ Have desire for sweets ☐ Feel hungry again soon after meal ☐ Need to snack between meals
ENERGY LEVELS	Normal energy response to meal: ☐ Energy is restored after eating ☐ Have good, lasting, "normal" sense of energy and well-being	Poor energy response to meal: ☐ Too much or too little energy ☐ Become hyper, jittery, shaky, nervous, or speedy ☐ Feel hyper, but exhausted "underneath" ☐ Energy drop, fatigue, exhaustion, sleepiness, drowsiness, lethargy, or listlessness
MENTAL EMOTIONAL WELL-BEING	Normal qualities: ☐ Improved well-being ☐ Sense of feeling refueled and restored ☐ Upliftment in emotions ☐ Improved clarity and acuity of mind ☐ Normalization of thought processes	Abnormal qualities: ☐ Mentally slow, sluggish, spacey ☐ Inability to think quickly or clearly ☐ Hyper, overly rapid thoughts ☐ Inability to focus/hold attention ☐ Hypo traits: Apathy, depression, sadness ☐ Hyper traits: Anxious, obsessive, fearful, angry, short tempered, or irritable, etc.

DIET AND EXERCISE JOURNAL   WEEK 9 / DAY 62

Date : _____

Diet and Exercise Goals : _____

_____

_____

_____

_____

Meal	List of Food You Ate	Additional Notes
Breakfast		
Lunch		
Dinner		
Snack		

	Exercises	Duration, Repetitions and Additional Notes
Body Balancing Streches		
Core Stability Exercises		
Body Allignment Exercises		

Nothing is likely to help a person overcome or endure troubles than the consciousness
of having a task in life. - Victor Frankl

Diet Record Sheet	☐Breakfast	☐Lunch	☐Dinner
Reactions after a meal	**Good**		**Bad**
APPETITE FULLNESS / SATISFACTION SWEET CRAVINGS	Following the meal . . . ☐ Feel full, satisfied ☐ Do NOT have sweet cravings ☐ Do NOT desire more food ☐ Do NOT get hungry soon after ☐ Do NOT need to snack before next meal		Following the meal . . . ☐ Feel physically full, but still hungry ☐ Don't feel satisfied; feel like something was missing from meal ☐ Have desire for sweets ☐ Feel hungry again soon after meal ☐ Need to snack between meals
ENERGY LEVELS	Normal energy response to meal: ☐ Energy is restored after eating ☐ Have good, lasting, "normal" sense of energy and well-being		Poor energy response to meal: ☐ Too much or too little energy ☐ Become hyper, jittery, shaky, nervous, or speedy ☐ Feel hyper, but exhausted "underneath" ☐ Energy drop, fatigue, exhaustion, sleepiness, drowsiness, lethargy, or listlessness
MENTAL EMOTIONAL WELL-BEING	Normal qualities: ☐ Improved well-being ☐ Sense of feeling refueled and restored ☐ Upliftment in emotions ☐ Improved clarity and acuity of mind ☐ Normalization of thought processes		Abnormal qualities: ☐ Mentally slow, sluggish, spacey ☐ Inability to think quickly or clearly ☐ Hyper, overly rapid thoughts ☐ Inability to focus/hold attention ☐ Hypo traits: Apathy, depression, sadness ☐ Hyper traits: Anxious, obsessive, fearful, angry, short tempered, or irritable, etc.

DIET AND EXERCISE JOURNAL

WEEK 9 / DAY 63

Date : _____

Diet and Exercise Goals : _____

_____

_____

_____

_____

Meal	List of Food You Ate	Additional Notes
Breakfast		
Lunch		
Dinner		
Snack		

	Exercises	Duration, Repetitions and Additional Notes
Body Balancing Streches		
Core Stability Exercises		
Body Allignment Exercises		

Courage is resistance to fear, mastery of fear - not absence of fear. - Mark Twain

Diet Record Sheet	☐Breakfast ☐Lunch ☐Dinner	
Reactions after a meal	**Good**	**Bad**
APPETITE FULLNESS / SATISFACTION SWEET CRAVINGS	Following the meal . . . ☐ Feel full, satisfied ☐ Do NOT have sweet cravings ☐ Do NOT desire more food ☐ Do NOT get hungry soon after ☐ Do NOT need to snack before next meal	Following the meal . . . ☐ Feel physically full, but still hungry ☐ Don't feel satisfied; feel like something was missing from meal ☐ Have desire for sweets ☐ Feel hungry again soon after meal ☐ Need to snack between meals
ENERGY LEVELS	Normal energy response to meal: ☐ Energy is restored after eating ☐ Have good, lasting, "normal" sense of energy and well-being	Poor energy response to meal: ☐ Too much or too little energy ☐ Become hyper, jittery, shaky, nervous, or speedy ☐ Feel hyper, but exhausted "underneath" ☐ Energy drop, fatigue, exhaustion, sleepiness, drowsiness, lethargy, or listlessness
MENTAL EMOTIONAL WELL-BEING	Normal qualities: ☐ Improved well-being ☐ Sense of feeling refueled and restored ☐ Upliftment in emotions ☐ Improved clarity and acuity of mind ☐ Normalization of thought processes	Abnormal qualities: ☐ Mentally slow, sluggish, spacey ☐ Inability to think quickly or clearly ☐ Hyper, overly rapid thoughts ☐ Inability to focus/hold attention ☐ Hypo traits: Apathy, depression, sadness ☐ Hyper traits: Anxious, obsessive, fearful, angry, short tempered, or irritable, etc.

DIET AND EXERCISE JOURNAL

WEEK 10 / DAY 64

Date : _____

Diet and Exercise Goals : _____

_____

_____

_____

_____

Meal	List of Food You Ate	Additional Notes
Breakfast		
Lunch		
Dinner		
Snack		

	Exercises	Duration, Repetitions and Additional Notes
Body Balancing Streches		
Core Stability Exercises		
Body Allignment Exercises		

"I don't know what's in the box, but I love it. Unopened gifts contain hope. " - Jarod Kintz

Diet Record Sheet	☐Breakfast ☐Lunch ☐Dinner	
Reactions after a meal	Good	Bad
APPETITE FULLNESS / SATISFACTION SWEET CRAVINGS	Following the meal . . . ☐ Feel full, satisfied ☐ Do NOT have sweet cravings ☐ Do NOT desire more food ☐ Do NOT get hungry soon after ☐ Do NOT need to snack before next meal	Following the meal . . . ☐ Feel physically full, but still hungry ☐ Don't feel satisfied; feel like something was missing from meal ☐ Have desire for sweets ☐ Feel hungry again soon after meal ☐ Need to snack between meals
ENERGY LEVELS	Normal energy response to meal: ☐ Energy is restored after eating ☐ Have good, lasting, "normal" sense of energy and well-being	Poor energy response to meal: ☐ Too much or too little energy ☐ Become hyper, jittery, shaky, nervous, or speedy ☐ Feel hyper, but exhausted "underneath" ☐ Energy drop, fatigue, exhaustion, sleepiness, drowsiness, lethargy, or listlessness
MENTAL EMOTIONAL WELL-BEING	Normal qualities: ☐ Improved well-being ☐ Sense of feeling refueled and restored ☐ Upliftment in emotions ☐ Improved clarity and acuity of mind ☐ Normalization of thought processes	Abnormal qualities: ☐ Mentally slow, sluggish, spacey ☐ Inability to think quickly or clearly ☐ Hyper, overly rapid thoughts ☐ Inability to focus/hold attention ☐ Hypo traits: Apathy, depression, sadness ☐ Hyper traits: Anxious, obsessive, fearful, angry, short tempered, or irritable, etc.

DIET AND EXERCISE JOURNAL　　　　　WEEK 10 / DAY 65

Date : _____

Diet and Exercise Goals : _____

_____

_____

_____

_____

Meal	List of Food You Ate	Additional Notes
Breakfast		
Lunch		
Dinner		
Snack		

	Exercises	Duration, Repetitions and Additional Notes
Body Balancing Streches		
Core Stability Exercises		
Body Allignment Exercises		

Courage doesn't always roar. Sometimes, courage is the quiet voice at the end of the day saying,
"I will try again tomorrow". - Mary Anne Radmacher

Diet Record Sheet	☐Breakfast ☐Lunch ☐Dinner	
Reactions after a meal	Good	Bad
APPETITE FULLNESS / SATISFACTION SWEET CRAVINGS	Following the meal . . . ☐ Feel full, satisfied ☐ Do NOT have sweet cravings ☐ Do NOT desire more food ☐ Do NOT get hungry soon after ☐ Do NOT need to snack before next meal	Following the meal . . . ☐ Feel physically full, but still hungry ☐ Don't feel satisfied; feel like something was missing from meal ☐ Have desire for sweets ☐ Feel hungry again soon after meal ☐ Need to snack between meals
ENERGY LEVELS	Normal energy response to meal: ☐ Energy is restored after eating ☐ Have good, lasting, "normal" sense of energy and well-being	Poor energy response to meal: ☐ Too much or too little energy ☐ Become hyper, jittery, shaky, nervous, or speedy ☐ Feel hyper, but exhausted "underneath" ☐ Energy drop, fatigue, exhaustion, sleepiness, drowsiness, lethargy, or listlessness
MENTAL EMOTIONAL WELL-BEING	Normal qualities: ☐ Improved well-being ☐ Sense of feeling refueled and restored ☐ Upliftment in emotions ☐ Improved clarity and acuity of mind ☐ Normalization of thought processes	Abnormal qualities: ☐ Mentally slow, sluggish, spacey ☐ Inability to think quickly or clearly ☐ Hyper, overly rapid thoughts ☐ Inability to focus/hold attention ☐ Hypo traits: Apathy, depression, sadness ☐ Hyper traits: Anxious, obsessive, fearful, angry, short tempered, or irritable, etc.

DIET AND EXERCISE JOURNAL

WEEK 10 / DAY 66

Date : _____

Diet and Exercise Goals : _____

_____

_____

_____

_____

Meal	List of Food You Ate	Additional Notes
Breakfast		
Lunch		
Dinner		
Snack		

	Exercises	Duration, Repetitions and Additional Notes
Body Balancing Streches		
Core Stability Exercises		
Body Allignment Exercises		

Any change, even a change for the better,
is always accompanied by drawbacks and discomforts. - Arnold Bennett

Diet Record Sheet	☐Breakfast ☐Lunch ☐Dinner	
Reactions after a meal	**Good**	**Bad**
APPETITE FULLNESS / SATISFACTION SWEET CRAVINGS	Following the meal . . . ☐ Feel full, satisfied ☐ Do NOT have sweet cravings ☐ Do NOT desire more food ☐ Do NOT get hungry soon after ☐ Do NOT need to snack before next meal	Following the meal . . . ☐ Feel physically full, but still hungry ☐ Don't feel satisfied; feel like something was missing from meal ☐ Have desire for sweets ☐ Feel hungry again soon after meal ☐ Need to snack between meals
ENERGY LEVELS	Normal energy response to meal: ☐ Energy is restored after eating ☐ Have good, lasting, "normal" sense of energy and well-being	Poor energy response to meal: ☐ Too much or too little energy ☐ Become hyper, jittery, shaky, nervous, or speedy ☐ Feel hyper, but exhausted "underneath" ☐ Energy drop, fatigue, exhaustion, sleepiness, drowsiness, lethargy, or listlessness
MENTAL EMOTIONAL WELL-BEING	Normal qualities: ☐ Improved well-being ☐ Sense of feeling refueled and restored ☐ Upliftment in emotions ☐ Improved clarity and acuity of mind ☐ Normalization of thought processes	Abnormal qualities: ☐ Mentally slow, sluggish, spacey ☐ Inability to think quickly or clearly ☐ Hyper, overly rapid thoughts ☐ Inability to focus/hold attention ☐ Hypo traits: Apathy, depression, sadness ☐ Hyper traits: Anxious, obsessive, fearful, angry, short tempered, or irritable, etc.

DIET AND EXERCISE JOURNAL   WEEK 10 / DAY 67

Date : _____

Diet and Exercise Goals : _____

_____

_____

_____

_____

Meal	List of Food You Ate	Additional Notes
Breakfast		
Lunch		
Dinner		
Snack		

	Exercises	Duration, Repetitions and Additional Notes
Body Balancing Streches		
Core Stability Exercises		
Body Allignment Exercises		

> "I hated every minute of training, but I said, 'Don't quit.
> Suffer now and live the rest of your life as a champion." - Muhammad Ali

Diet Record Sheet	☐Breakfast ☐Lunch ☐Dinner	
Reactions after a meal	Good	Bad
APPETITE FULLNESS / SATISFACTION SWEET CRAVINGS	Following the meal . . . ☐ Feel full, satisfied ☐ Do NOT have sweet cravings ☐ Do NOT desire more food ☐ Do NOT get hungry soon after ☐ Do NOT need to snack before next meal	Following the meal . . . ☐ Feel physically full, but still hungry ☐ Don't feel satisfied; feel like something was missing from meal ☐ Have desire for sweets ☐ Feel hungry again soon after meal ☐ Need to snack between meals
ENERGY LEVELS	Normal energy response to meal: ☐ Energy is restored after eating ☐ Have good, lasting, "normal" sense of energy and well-being	Poor energy response to meal: ☐ Too much or too little energy ☐ Become hyper, jittery, shaky, nervous, or speedy ☐ Feel hyper, but exhausted "underneath" ☐ Energy drop, fatigue, exhaustion, sleepiness, drowsiness, lethargy, or listlessness
MENTAL EMOTIONAL WELL-BEING	Normal qualities: ☐ Improved well-being ☐ Sense of feeling refueled and restored ☐ Upliftment in emotions ☐ Improved clarity and acuity of mind ☐ Normalization of thought processes	Abnormal qualities: ☐ Mentally slow, sluggish, spacey ☐ Inability to think quickly or clearly ☐ Hyper, overly rapid thoughts ☐ Inability to focus/hold attention ☐ Hypo traits: Apathy, depression, sadness ☐ Hyper traits: Anxious, obsessive, fearful, angry, short tempered, or irritable, etc.

DIET AND EXERCISE JOURNAL

WEEK 10 / DAY 68

Date : _____

Diet and Exercise Goals : _____

_____

_____

_____

_____

Meal	List of Food You Ate	Additional Notes
Breakfast		
Lunch		
Dinner		
Snack		

	Exercises	Duration, Repetitions and Additional Notes
Body Balancing Streches		
Core Stability Exercises		
Body Allignment Exercises		

The bad days have two things in common: you know the right thing to do,
and you let someone talk you out of doing it - Tom Bihn

Diet Record Sheet	☐Breakfast ☐Lunch ☐Dinner	
Reactions after a meal	**Good**	**Bad**
APPETITE FULLNESS / SATISFACTION SWEET CRAVINGS	Following the meal . . . ☐ Feel full, satisfied ☐ Do NOT have sweet cravings ☐ Do NOT desire more food ☐ Do NOT get hungry soon after ☐ Do NOT need to snack before next meal	Following the meal . . . ☐ Feel physically full, but still hungry ☐ Don't feel satisfied; feel like something was missing from meal ☐ Have desire for sweets ☐ Feel hungry again soon after meal ☐ Need to snack between meals
ENERGY LEVELS	Normal energy response to meal: ☐ Energy is restored after eating ☐ Have good, lasting, "normal" sense of energy and well-being	Poor energy response to meal: ☐ Too much or too little energy ☐ Become hyper, jittery, shaky, nervous, or speedy ☐ Feel hyper, but exhausted "underneath" ☐ Energy drop, fatigue, exhaustion, sleepiness, drowsiness, lethargy, or listlessness
MENTAL EMOTIONAL WELL-BEING	Normal qualities: ☐ Improved well-being ☐ Sense of feeling refueled and restored ☐ Upliftment in emotions ☐ Improved clarity and acuity of mind ☐ Normalization of thought processes	Abnormal qualities: ☐ Mentally slow, sluggish, spacey ☐ Inability to think quickly or clearly ☐ Hyper, overly rapid thoughts ☐ Inability to focus/hold attention ☐ Hypo traits: Apathy, depression, sadness ☐ Hyper traits: Anxious, obsessive, fearful, angry, short tempered, or irritable, etc.

DIET AND EXERCISE JOURNAL

Date : _____

Diet and Exercise Goals : _____

_____

_____

_____

_____

_____

Meal	List of Food You Ate	Additional Notes
Breakfast		
Lunch		
Dinner		
Snack		

	Exercises	Duration, Repetitions and Additional Notes
Body Balancing Streches		
Core Stability Exercises		
Body Allignment Exercises		

Pain is inevitable. Suffering is optional - Anony-mouse

Diet Record Sheet	☐Breakfast ☐Lunch ☐Dinner	
Reactions after a meal	**Good**	**Bad**
APPETITE FULLNESS / SATISFACTION SWEET CRAVINGS	Following the meal . . . ☐ Feel full, satisfied ☐ Do NOT have sweet cravings ☐ Do NOT desire more food ☐ Do NOT get hungry soon after ☐ Do NOT need to snack before next meal	Following the meal . . . ☐ Feel physically full, but still hungry ☐ Don't feel satisfied; feel like something was missing from meal ☐ Have desire for sweets ☐ Feel hungry again soon after meal ☐ Need to snack between meals
ENERGY LEVELS	Normal energy response to meal: ☐ Energy is restored after eating ☐ Have good, lasting, "normal" sense of energy and well-being	Poor energy response to meal: ☐ Too much or too little energy ☐ Become hyper, jittery, shaky, nervous, or speedy ☐ Feel hyper, but exhausted "underneath" ☐ Energy drop, fatigue, exhaustion, sleepiness, drowsiness, lethargy, or listlessness
MENTAL EMOTIONAL WELL-BEING	Normal qualities: ☐ Improved well-being ☐ Sense of feeling refueled and restored ☐ Upliftment in emotions ☐ Improved clarity and acuity of mind ☐ Normalization of thought processes	Abnormal qualities: ☐ Mentally slow, sluggish, spacey ☐ Inability to think quickly or clearly ☐ Hyper, overly rapid thoughts ☐ Inability to focus/hold attention ☐ Hypo traits: Apathy, depression, sadness ☐ Hyper traits: Anxious, obsessive, fearful, angry, short tempered, or irritable, etc.

DIET AND EXERCISE JOURNAL   WEEK 10 / DAY 70

Date : _____

Diet and Exercise Goals : _____

_____

_____

_____

_____

Meal	List of Food You Ate	Additional Notes
Breakfast		
Lunch		
Dinner		
Snack		

	Exercises	Duration, Repetitions and Additional Notes
Body Balancing Streches		
Core Stability Exercises		
Body Allignment Exercises		

You gain strength, courage and confidence by every experience in which
you really stop to look fear in the face - Eleanor Roosevelt

Diet Record Sheet	☐Breakfast ☐Lunch ☐Dinner	
Reactions after a meal	**Good**	**Bad**
APPETITE FULLNESS / SATISFACTION SWEET CRAVINGS	Following the meal . . . ☐ Feel full, satisfied ☐ Do NOT have sweet cravings ☐ Do NOT desire more food ☐ Do NOT get hungry soon after ☐ Do NOT need to snack before next meal	Following the meal . . . ☐ Feel physically full, but still hungry ☐ Don't feel satisfied; feel like something was missing from meal ☐ Have desire for sweets ☐ Feel hungry again soon after meal ☐ Need to snack between meals
ENERGY LEVELS	Normal energy response to meal: ☐ Energy is restored after eating ☐ Have good, lasting, "normal" sense of energy and well-being	Poor energy response to meal: ☐ Too much or too little energy ☐ Become hyper, jittery, shaky, nervous, or speedy ☐ Feel hyper, but exhausted "underneath" ☐ Energy drop, fatigue, exhaustion, sleepiness, drowsiness, lethargy, or listlessness
MENTAL EMOTIONAL WELL-BEING	Normal qualities: ☐ Improved well-being ☐ Sense of feeling refueled and restored ☐ Upliftment in emotions ☐ Improved clarity and acuity of mind ☐ Normalization of thought processes	Abnormal qualities: ☐ Mentally slow, sluggish, spacey ☐ Inability to think quickly or clearly ☐ Hyper, overly rapid thoughts ☐ Inability to focus/hold attention ☐ Hypo traits: Apathy, depression, sadness ☐ Hyper traits: Anxious, obsessive, fearful, angry, short tempered, or irritable, etc.

DIET AND EXERCISE JOURNAL

WEEK 11 / DAY 71

Date : _____

Diet and Exercise Goals : _____

_____

_____

_____

_____

Meal	List of Food You Ate	Additional Notes
Breakfast		
Lunch		
Dinner		
Snack		

	Exercises	Duration, Repetitions and Additional Notes
Body Balancing Streches		
Core Stability Exercises		
Body Allignment Exercises		

Do one thing every day that scares you. - Eleanor Roosevelt.

198

Diet Record Sheet	☐Breakfast ☐Lunch ☐Dinner	
Reactions after a meal	**Good**	**Bad**
APPETITE FULLNESS / SATISFACTION SWEET CRAVINGS	Following the meal . . . ☐ Feel full, satisfied ☐ Do NOT have sweet cravings ☐ Do NOT desire more food ☐ Do NOT get hungry soon after ☐ Do NOT need to snack before next meal	Following the meal . . . ☐ Feel physically full, but still hungry ☐ Don't feel satisfied; feel like something was missing from meal ☐ Have desire for sweets ☐ Feel hungry again soon after meal ☐ Need to snack between meals
ENERGY LEVELS	Normal energy response to meal: ☐ Energy is restored after eating ☐ Have good, lasting, "normal" sense of energy and well-being	Poor energy response to meal: ☐ Too much or too little energy ☐ Become hyper, jittery, shaky, nervous, or speedy ☐ Feel hyper, but exhausted "underneath" ☐ Energy drop, fatigue, exhaustion, sleepiness, drowsiness, lethargy, or listlessness
MENTAL EMOTIONAL WELL-BEING	Normal qualities: ☐ Improved well-being ☐ Sense of feeling refueled and restored ☐ Upliftment in emotions ☐ Improved clarity and acuity of mind ☐ Normalization of thought processes	Abnormal qualities: ☐ Mentally slow, sluggish, spacey ☐ Inability to think quickly or clearly ☐ Hyper, overly rapid thoughts ☐ Inability to focus/hold attention ☐ Hypo traits: Apathy, depression, sadness ☐ Hyper traits: Anxious, obsessive, fearful, angry, short tempered, or irritable, etc.

DIET AND EXERCISE JOURNAL   WEEK 11 / DAY 72

Date : _____

Diet and Exercise Goals : _____

_____

_____

_____

_____

Meal	List of Food You Ate	Additional Notes
Breakfast		
Lunch		
Dinner		
Snack		

	Exercises	Duration, Repetitions and Additional Notes
Body Balancing Streches		
Core Stability Exercises		
Body Allignment Exercises		

If you cannot do great things, do small things in a great way. - Napoleon Hill

Diet Record Sheet		☐Breakfast ☐Lunch ☐Dinner
Reactions after a meal	Good	Bad
APPETITE FULLNESS / SATISFACTION SWEET CRAVINGS	Following the meal . . . ☐ Feel full, satisfied ☐ Do NOT have sweet cravings ☐ Do NOT desire more food ☐ Do NOT get hungry soon after ☐ Do NOT need to snack before next meal	Following the meal . . . ☐ Feel physically full, but still hungry ☐ Don't feel satisfied; feel like something was missing from meal ☐ Have desire for sweets ☐ Feel hungry again soon after meal ☐ Need to snack between meals
ENERGY LEVELS	Normal energy response to meal: ☐ Energy is restored after eating ☐ Have good, lasting, "normal" sense of energy and well-being	Poor energy response to meal: ☐ Too much or too little energy ☐ Become hyper, jittery, shaky, nervous, or speedy ☐ Feel hyper, but exhausted "underneath" ☐ Energy drop, fatigue, exhaustion, sleepiness, drowsiness, lethargy, or listlessness
MENTAL EMOTIONAL WELL-BEING	Normal qualities: ☐ Improved well-being ☐ Sense of feeling refueled and restored ☐ Upliftment in emotions ☐ Improved clarity and acuity of mind ☐ Normalization of thought processes	Abnormal qualities: ☐ Mentally slow, sluggish, spacey ☐ Inability to think quickly or clearly ☐ Hyper, overly rapid thoughts ☐ Inability to focus/hold attention ☐ Hypo traits: Apathy, depression, sadness ☐ Hyper traits: Anxious, obsessive, fearful, angry, short tempered, or irritable, etc.

DIET AND EXERCISE JOURNAL   WEEK 11 / DAY 73

Date : _____

Diet and Exercise Goals : _____

_____

_____

_____

_____

Meal	List of Food You Ate	Additional Notes
Breakfast		
Lunch		
Dinner		
Snack		

	Exercises	Duration, Repetitions and Additional Notes
Body Balancing Streches		
Core Stability Exercises		
Body Allignment Exercises		

What you do makes a difference,
and you have to decide what kind of difference you want to make. - Jane Goodall

Diet Record Sheet		☐Breakfast ☐Lunch ☐Dinner
Reactions after a meal	Good	Bad
APPETITE FULLNESS / SATISFACTION SWEET CRAVINGS	Following the meal . . . ☐ Feel full, satisfied ☐ Do NOT have sweet cravings ☐ Do NOT desire more food ☐ Do NOT get hungry soon after ☐ Do NOT need to snack before next meal	Following the meal . . . ☐ Feel physically full, but still hungry ☐ Don't feel satisfied; feel like something was missing from meal ☐ Have desire for sweets ☐ Feel hungry again soon after meal ☐ Need to snack between meals
ENERGY LEVELS	Normal energy response to meal: ☐ Energy is restored after eating ☐ Have good, lasting, "normal" sense of energy and well-being	Poor energy response to meal: ☐ Too much or too little energy ☐ Become hyper, jittery, shaky, nervous, or speedy ☐ Feel hyper, but exhausted "underneath" ☐ Energy drop, fatigue, exhaustion, sleepiness, drowsiness, lethargy, or listlessness
MENTAL EMOTIONAL WELL-BEING	Normal qualities: ☐ Improved well-being ☐ Sense of feeling refueled and restored ☐ Upliftment in emotions ☐ Improved clarity and acuity of mind ☐ Normalization of thought processes	Abnormal qualities: ☐ Mentally slow, sluggish, spacey ☐ Inability to think quickly or clearly ☐ Hyper, overly rapid thoughts ☐ Inability to focus/hold attention ☐ Hypo traits: Apathy, depression, sadness ☐ Hyper traits: Anxious, obsessive, fearful, angry, short tempered, or irritable, etc.

DIET AND EXERCISE JOURNAL   WEEK 11 / DAY 74

Date : _____

Diet and Exercise Goals : _____

_____

_____

_____

_____

Meal	List of Food You Ate	Additional Notes
Breakfast		
Lunch		
Dinner		
Snack		

	Exercises	Duration, Repetitions and Additional Notes
Body Balancing Streches		
Core Stability Exercises		
Body Allignment Exercises		

Do you want to know who you are? Don't ask. Act! Action will delineate and define you. - Thomas Jefferson

Diet Record Sheet	☐Breakfast	☐Lunch	☐Dinner

Reactions after a meal	Good	Bad
APPETITE FULLNESS / SATISFACTION SWEET CRAVINGS	Following the meal . . . ☐ Feel full, satisfied ☐ Do NOT have sweet cravings ☐ Do NOT desire more food ☐ Do NOT get hungry soon after ☐ Do NOT need to snack before next meal	Following the meal . . . ☐ Feel physically full, but still hungry ☐ Don't feel satisfied; feel like something was missing from meal ☐ Have desire for sweets ☐ Feel hungry again soon after meal ☐ Need to snack between meals
ENERGY LEVELS	Normal energy response to meal: ☐ Energy is restored after eating ☐ Have good, lasting, "normal" sense of energy and well-being	Poor energy response to meal: ☐ Too much or too little energy ☐ Become hyper, jittery, shaky, nervous, or speedy ☐ Feel hyper, but exhausted "underneath" ☐ Energy drop, fatigue, exhaustion, sleepiness, drowsiness, lethargy, or listlessness
MENTAL EMOTIONAL WELL-BEING	Normal qualities: ☐ Improved well-being ☐ Sense of feeling refueled and restored ☐ Upliftment in emotions ☐ Improved clarity and acuity of mind ☐ Normalization of thought processes	Abnormal qualities: ☐ Mentally slow, sluggish, spacey ☐ Inability to think quickly or clearly ☐ Hyper, overly rapid thoughts ☐ Inability to focus/hold attention ☐ Hypo traits: Apathy, depression, sadness ☐ Hyper traits: Anxious, obsessive, fearful, angry, short tempered, or irritable, etc.

DIET AND EXERCISE JOURNAL   WEEK 11 / DAY 75

Date : _____

Diet and Exercise Goals : _____

_____

_____

_____

_____

Meal	List of Food You Ate	Additional Notes
Breakfast		
Lunch		
Dinner		
Snack		

	Exercises	Duration, Repetitions and Additional Notes
Body Balancing Streches		
Core Stability Exercises		
Body Allignment Exercises		

A day without laughter is a day wasted. - Charles Chaplin

Diet Record Sheet	☐Breakfast ☐Lunch ☐Dinner	
Reactions after a meal	Good	Bad
APPETITE FULLNESS / SATISFACTION SWEET CRAVINGS	Following the meal . . . ☐ Feel full, satisfied ☐ Do NOT have sweet cravings ☐ Do NOT desire more food ☐ Do NOT get hungry soon after ☐ Do NOT need to snack before next meal	Following the meal . . . ☐ Feel physically full, but still hungry ☐ Don't feel satisfied; feel like something was missing from meal ☐ Have desire for sweets ☐ Feel hungry again soon after meal ☐ Need to snack between meals
ENERGY LEVELS	Normal energy response to meal: ☐ Energy is restored after eating ☐ Have good, lasting, "normal" sense of energy and well-being	Poor energy response to meal: ☐ Too much or too little energy ☐ Become hyper, jittery, shaky, nervous, or speedy ☐ Feel hyper, but exhausted "underneath" ☐ Energy drop, fatigue, exhaustion, sleepiness, drowsiness, lethargy, or listlessness
MENTAL EMOTIONAL WELL-BEING	Normal qualities: ☐ Improved well-being ☐ Sense of feeling refueled and restored ☐ Upliftment in emotions ☐ Improved clarity and acuity of mind ☐ Normalization of thought processes	Abnormal qualities: ☐ Mentally slow, sluggish, spacey ☐ Inability to think quickly or clearly ☐ Hyper, overly rapid thoughts ☐ Inability to focus/hold attention ☐ Hypo traits: Apathy, depression, sadness ☐ Hyper traits: Anxious, obsessive, fearful, angry, short tempered, or irritable, etc.

DIET AND EXERCISE JOURNAL

WEEK 11 / DAY 76

Date : _____

Diet and Exercise Goals : _____

_____

_____

_____

_____

Meal	List of Food You Ate	Additional Notes
Breakfast		
Lunch		
Dinner		
Snack		

	Exercises	Duration, Repetitions and Additional Notes
Body Balancing Streches		
Core Stability Exercises		
Body Allignment Exercises		

Ignore those that make you fearful and sad, that degrade you back towards disease and death. – Rumi

Diet Record Sheet	☐Breakfast ☐Lunch ☐Dinner	
Reactions after a meal	Good	Bad
APPETITE FULLNESS / SATISFACTION SWEET CRAVINGS	Following the meal . . . ☐ Feel full, satisfied ☐ Do NOT have sweet cravings ☐ Do NOT desire more food ☐ Do NOT get hungry soon after ☐ Do NOT need to snack before next meal	Following the meal . . . ☐ Feel physically full, but still hungry ☐ Don't feel satisfied; feel like something was missing from meal ☐ Have desire for sweets ☐ Feel hungry again soon after meal ☐ Need to snack between meals
ENERGY LEVELS	Normal energy response to meal: ☐ Energy is restored after eating ☐ Have good, lasting, "normal" sense of energy and well-being	Poor energy response to meal: ☐ Too much or too little energy ☐ Become hyper, jittery, shaky, nervous, or speedy ☐ Feel hyper, but exhausted "underneath" ☐ Energy drop, fatigue, exhaustion, sleepiness, drowsiness, lethargy, or listlessness
MENTAL EMOTIONAL WELL-BEING	Normal qualities: ☐ Improved well-being ☐ Sense of feeling refueled and restored ☐ Upliftment in emotions ☐ Improved clarity and acuity of mind ☐ Normalization of thought processes	Abnormal qualities: ☐ Mentally slow, sluggish, spacey ☐ Inability to think quickly or clearly ☐ Hyper, overly rapid thoughts ☐ Inability to focus/hold attention ☐ Hypo traits: Apathy, depression, sadness ☐ Hyper traits: Anxious, obsessive, fearful, angry, short tempered, or irritable, etc.

DIET AND EXERCISE JOURNAL
WEEK 11 / DAY 77

Date : _____

Diet and Exercise Goals : _____

_____

_____

_____

_____

Meal	List of Food You Ate	Additional Notes
Breakfast		
Lunch		
Dinner		
Snack		

	Exercises	Duration, Repetitions and Additional Notes
Body Balancing Streches		
Core Stability Exercises		
Body Allignment Exercises		

Risks must be taken because the greatest hazard in life is to risk nothing. - Leo Buscaglia

Diet Record Sheet	□Breakfast □Lunch □Dinner	
Reactions after a meal	Good	Bad
APPETITE FULLNESS / SATISFACTION SWEET CRAVINGS	Following the meal . . . ☐ Feel full, satisfied ☐ Do NOT have sweet cravings ☐ Do NOT desire more food ☐ Do NOT get hungry soon after ☐ Do NOT need to snack before next meal	Following the meal . . . ☐ Feel physically full, but still hungry ☐ Don't feel satisfied; feel like something was missing from meal ☐ Have desire for sweets ☐ Feel hungry again soon after meal ☐ Need to snack between meals
ENERGY LEVELS	Normal energy response to meal: ☐ Energy is restored after eating ☐ Have good, lasting, "normal" sense of energy and well-being	Poor energy response to meal: ☐ Too much or too little energy ☐ Become hyper, jittery, shaky, nervous, or speedy ☐ Feel hyper, but exhausted "underneath" ☐ Energy drop, fatigue, exhaustion, sleepiness, drowsiness, lethargy, or listlessness
MENTAL EMOTIONAL WELL-BEING	Normal qualities: ☐ Improved well-being ☐ Sense of feeling refueled and restored ☐ Upliftment in emotions ☐ Improved clarity and acuity of mind ☐ Normalization of thought processes	Abnormal qualities: ☐ Mentally slow, sluggish, spacey ☐ Inability to think quickly or clearly ☐ Hyper, overly rapid thoughts ☐ Inability to focus/hold attention ☐ Hypo traits: Apathy, depression, sadness ☐ Hyper traits: Anxious, obsessive, fearful, angry, short tempered, or irritable, etc.

Week 12: Scoliosis Symptoms Review

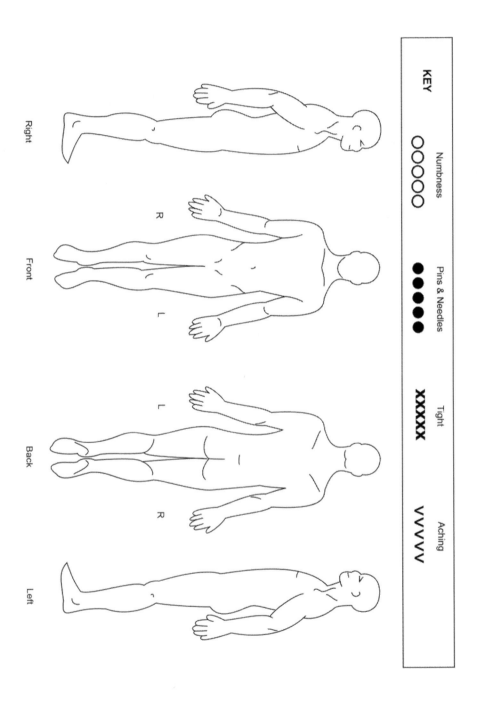

Week 12: Trigger Point Mapping

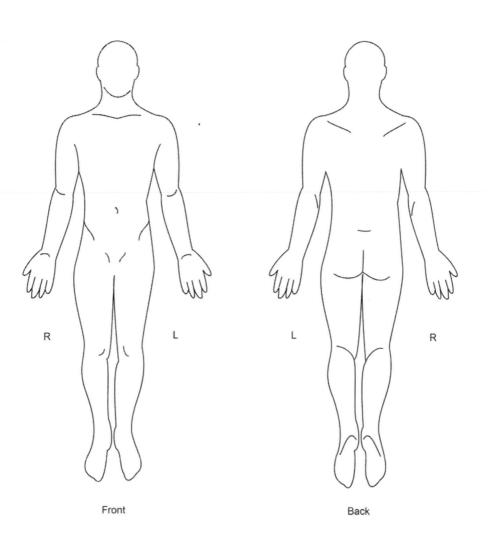

Front   Back

DIET AND EXERCISE JOURNAL   WEEK 12 / DAY 78

Date : _____

Diet and Exercise Goals : _____

_____

_____

_____

_____

_____

Meal	List of Food You Ate	Additional Notes
Breakfast		
Lunch		
Dinner		
Snack		

	Exercises	Duration, Repetitions and Additional Notes
Body Balancing Streches		
Core Stability Exercises		
Body Allignment Exercises		

There is no dishonor in losing the race.
There is only dishonor in not racing because you are afraid to lose. - Garth Stein

Diet Record Sheet	□Breakfast	□Lunch	□Dinner
Reactions after a meal	**Good**		**Bad**
APPETITE FULLNESS / SATISFACTION SWEET CRAVINGS	Following the meal . . . □ Feel full, satisfied □ Do NOT have sweet cravings □ Do NOT desire more food □ Do NOT get hungry soon after □ Do NOT need to snack before next meal		Following the meal . . . □ Feel physically full, but still hungry □ Don't feel satisfied; feel like something was missing from meal □ Have desire for sweets □ Feel hungry again soon after meal □ Need to snack between meals
ENERGY LEVELS	Normal energy response to meal: □ Energy is restored after eating □ Have good, lasting, "normal" sense of energy and well-being		Poor energy response to meal: □ Too much or too little energy □ Become hyper, jittery, shaky, nervous, or speedy □ Feel hyper, but exhausted "underneath" □ Energy drop, fatigue, exhaustion, sleepiness, drowsiness, lethargy, or listlessness
MENTAL EMOTIONAL WELL-BEING	Normal qualities: □ Improved well-being □ Sense of feeling refueled and restored □ Upliftment in emotions □ Improved clarity and acuity of mind □ Normalization of thought processes		Abnormal qualities: □ Mentally slow, sluggish, spacey □ Inability to think quickly or clearly □ Hyper, overly rapid thoughts □ Inability to focus/hold attention □ Hypo traits: Apathy, depression, sadness □ Hyper traits: Anxious, obsessive, fearful, angry, short tempered, or irritable, etc.

DIET AND EXERCISE JOURNAL　　　　　　　WEEK 12 / DAY 79

Date : _____

Diet and Exercise Goals : _____

_____

_____

_____

_____

Meal	List of Food You Ate	Additional Notes
Breakfast		
Lunch		
Dinner		
Snack		

	Exercises	Duration, Repetitions and Additional Notes
Body Balancing Streches		
Core Stability Exercises		
Body Allignment Exercises		

The only person who can pull me down is myself,
and I'm not going to let myself pull me down anymore. - C. JoyBell C.

Diet Record Sheet	☐Breakfast ☐Lunch ☐Dinner	
Reactions after a meal	Good	Bad
APPETITE FULLNESS / SATISFACTION SWEET CRAVINGS	Following the meal . . . ☐ Feel full, satisfied ☐ Do NOT have sweet cravings ☐ Do NOT desire more food ☐ Do NOT get hungry soon after ☐ Do NOT need to snack before next meal	Following the meal . . . ☐ Feel physically full, but still hungry ☐ Don't feel satisfied; feel like something was missing from meal ☐ Have desire for sweets ☐ Feel hungry again soon after meal ☐ Need to snack between meals
ENERGY LEVELS	Normal energy response to meal: ☐ Energy is restored after eating ☐ Have good, lasting, "normal" sense of energy and well-being	Poor energy response to meal: ☐ Too much or too little energy ☐ Become hyper, jittery, shaky, nervous, or speedy ☐ Feel hyper, but exhausted "underneath" ☐ Energy drop, fatigue, exhaustion, sleepiness, drowsiness, lethargy, or listlessness
MENTAL EMOTIONAL WELL-BEING	Normal qualities: ☐ Improved well-being ☐ Sense of feeling refueled and restored ☐ Upliftment in emotions ☐ Improved clarity and acuity of mind ☐ Normalization of thought processes	Abnormal qualities: ☐ Mentally slow, sluggish, spacey ☐ Inability to think quickly or clearly ☐ Hyper, overly rapid thoughts ☐ Inability to focus/hold attention ☐ Hypo traits: Apathy, depression, sadness ☐ Hyper traits: Anxious, obsessive, fearful, angry, short tempered, or irritable, etc.

DIET AND EXERCISE JOURNAL   WEEK 12 / DAY 80

Date : _____

Diet and Exercise Goals : _____

_____

_____

_____

_____

Meal	List of Food You Ate	Additional Notes
Breakfast		
Lunch		
Dinner		
Snack		

	Exercises	Duration, Repetitions and Additional Notes
Body Balancing Streches		
Core Stability Exercises		
Body Allignment Exercises		

However mean your life is, meet it and live it. - Henry David Thoreau

218

Diet Record Sheet		☐Breakfast ☐Lunch ☐Dinner
Reactions after a meal	**Good**	**Bad**
APPETITE FULLNESS / SATISFACTION SWEET CRAVINGS	Following the meal . . . ☐ Feel full, satisfied ☐ Do NOT have sweet cravings ☐ Do NOT desire more food ☐ Do NOT get hungry soon after ☐ Do NOT need to snack before next meal	Following the meal . . . ☐ Feel physically full, but still hungry ☐ Don't feel satisfied; feel like something was missing from meal ☐ Have desire for sweets ☐ Feel hungry again soon after meal ☐ Need to snack between meals
ENERGY LEVELS	Normal energy response to meal: ☐ Energy is restored after eating ☐ Have good, lasting, "normal" sense of energy and well-being	Poor energy response to meal: ☐ Too much or too little energy ☐ Become hyper, jittery, shaky, nervous, or speedy ☐ Feel hyper, but exhausted "underneath" ☐ Energy drop, fatigue, exhaustion, sleepiness, drowsiness, lethargy, or listlessness
MENTAL EMOTIONAL WELL-BEING	Normal qualities: ☐ Improved well-being ☐ Sense of feeling refueled and restored ☐ Upliftment in emotions ☐ Improved clarity and acuity of mind ☐ Normalization of thought processes	Abnormal qualities: ☐ Mentally slow, sluggish, spacey ☐ Inability to think quickly or clearly ☐ Hyper, overly rapid thoughts ☐ Inability to focus/hold attention ☐ Hypo traits: Apathy, depression, sadness ☐ Hyper traits: Anxious, obsessive, fearful, angry, short tempered, or irritable, etc.

DIET AND EXERCISE JOURNAL   WEEK 12 / DAY 81

Date : _____

Diet and Exercise Goals : _____

_____

_____

_____

_____

Meal	List of Food You Ate	Additional Notes
Breakfast		
Lunch		
Dinner		
Snack		

	Exercises	Duration, Repetitions and Additional Notes
Body Balancing Streches		
Core Stability Exercises		
Body Allignment Exercises		

Success is not final, failure is not fatal: it is the courage to continue that counts. - Winston S. Churchill

Diet Record Sheet	☐Breakfast ☐Lunch ☐Dinner	
Reactions after a meal	**Good**	**Bad**
APPETITE FULLNESS / SATISFACTION SWEET CRAVINGS	Following the meal . . . ☐ Feel full, satisfied ☐ Do NOT have sweet cravings ☐ Do NOT desire more food ☐ Do NOT get hungry soon after ☐ Do NOT need to snack before next meal	Following the meal . . . ☐ Feel physically full, but still hungry ☐ Don't feel satisfied; feel like something was missing from meal ☐ Have desire for sweets ☐ Feel hungry again soon after meal ☐ Need to snack between meals
ENERGY LEVELS	Normal energy response to meal: ☐ Energy is restored after eating ☐ Have good, lasting, "normal" sense of energy and well-being	Poor energy response to meal: ☐ Too much or too little energy ☐ Become hyper, jittery, shaky, nervous, or speedy ☐ Feel hyper, but exhausted "underneath" ☐ Energy drop, fatigue, exhaustion, sleepiness, drowsiness, lethargy, or listlessness
MENTAL EMOTIONAL WELL-BEING	Normal qualities: ☐ Improved well-being ☐ Sense of feeling refueled and restored ☐ Upliftment in emotions ☐ Improved clarity and acuity of mind ☐ Normalization of thought processes	Abnormal qualities: ☐ Mentally slow, sluggish, spacey ☐ Inability to think quickly or clearly ☐ Hyper, overly rapid thoughts ☐ Inability to focus/hold attention ☐ Hypo traits: Apathy, depression, sadness ☐ Hyper traits: Anxious, obsessive, fearful, angry, short tempered, or irritable, etc.

DIET AND EXERCISE JOURNAL

WEEK 12 / DAY 82

Date : _____

Diet and Exercise Goals : _____

_____

_____

_____

_____

Meal	List of Food You Ate	Additional Notes
Breakfast		
Lunch		
Dinner		
Snack		

	Exercises	Duration, Repetitions and Additional Notes
Body Balancing Streches		
Core Stability Exercises		
Body Allignment Exercises		

At the end of the day, let there be no excuses, no explanations, no regrets. - Steve Maraboli

Diet Record Sheet	□Breakfast □Lunch □Dinner	
Reactions after a meal	**Good**	**Bad**
APPETITE FULLNESS / SATISFACTION SWEET CRAVINGS	Following the meal . . . ☐ Feel full, satisfied ☐ Do NOT have sweet cravings ☐ Do NOT desire more food ☐ Do NOT get hungry soon after ☐ Do NOT need to snack before next meal	Following the meal . . . ☐ Feel physically full, but still hungry ☐ Don't feel satisfied; feel like something was missing from meal ☐ Have desire for sweets ☐ Feel hungry again soon after meal ☐ Need to snack between meals
ENERGY LEVELS	Normal energy response to meal: ☐ Energy is restored after eating ☐ Have good, lasting, "normal" sense of energy and well-being	Poor energy response to meal: ☐ Too much or too little energy ☐ Become hyper, jittery, shaky, nervous, or speedy ☐ Feel hyper, but exhausted "underneath" ☐ Energy drop, fatigue, exhaustion, sleepiness, drowsiness, lethargy, or listlessness
MENTAL EMOTIONAL WELL-BEING	Normal qualities: ☐ Improved well-being ☐ Sense of feeling refueled and restored ☐ Upliftment in emotions ☐ Improved clarity and acuity of mind ☐ Normalization of thought processes	Abnormal qualities: ☐ Mentally slow, sluggish, spacey ☐ Inability to think quickly or clearly ☐ Hyper, overly rapid thoughts ☐ Inability to focus/hold attention ☐ Hypo traits: Apathy, depression, sadness ☐ Hyper traits: Anxious, obsessive, fearful, angry, short tempered, or irritable, etc.

DIET AND EXERCISE JOURNAL   WEEK 12 / DAY 83

Date : _____

Diet and Exercise Goals : _____

_____

_____

_____

_____

Meal	List of Food You Ate	Additional Notes
Breakfast		
Lunch		
Dinner		
Snack		

	Exercises	Duration, Repetitions and Additional Notes
Body Balancing Streches		
Core Stability Exercises		
Body Allignment Exercises		

When you arise in the morning, think of what a precious privilege it is to be alive- to breathe, to think, to enjoy, to love-then make that day count! - Steve Maraboli, Life, the Truth, and Being Free

Diet Record Sheet	☐Breakfast ☐Lunch ☐Dinner	
Reactions after a meal	**Good**	**Bad**
APPETITE FULLNESS / SATISFACTION SWEET CRAVINGS	Following the meal . . . ☐ Feel full, satisfied ☐ Do NOT have sweet cravings ☐ Do NOT desire more food ☐ Do NOT get hungry soon after ☐ Do NOT need to snack before next meal	Following the meal . . . ☐ Feel physically full, but still hungry ☐ Don't feel satisfied; feel like something was missing from meal ☐ Have desire for sweets ☐ Feel hungry again soon after meal ☐ Need to snack between meals
ENERGY LEVELS	Normal energy response to meal: ☐ Energy is restored after eating ☐ Have good, lasting, "normal" sense of energy and well-being	Poor energy response to meal: ☐ Too much or too little energy ☐ Become hyper, jittery, shaky, nervous, or speedy ☐ Feel hyper, but exhausted "underneath" ☐ Energy drop, fatigue, exhaustion, sleepiness, drowsiness, lethargy, or listlessness
MENTAL EMOTIONAL WELL-BEING	Normal qualities: ☐ Improved well-being ☐ Sense of feeling refueled and restored ☐ Upliftment in emotions ☐ Improved clarity and acuity of mind ☐ Normalization of thought processes	Abnormal qualities: ☐ Mentally slow, sluggish, spacey ☐ Inability to think quickly or clearly ☐ Hyper, overly rapid thoughts ☐ Inability to focus/hold attention ☐ Hypo traits: Apathy, depression, sadness ☐ Hyper traits: Anxious, obsessive, fearful, angry, short tempered, or irritable, etc.

DIET AND EXERCISE JOURNAL   WEEK 12 / DAY 84

Date : _____

Diet and Exercise Goals : _____

_____

_____

_____

_____

Meal	List of Food You Ate	Additional Notes
Breakfast		
Lunch		
Dinner		
Snack		

	Exercises	Duration, Repetitions and Additional Notes
Body Balancing Streches		
Core Stability Exercises		
Body Allignment Exercises		

When we are tired, we are attacked by ideas we conquered long ago. - Friedrich Nietzsche

Diet Record Sheet	☐Breakfast	☐Lunch	☐Dinner
Reactions after a meal	Good		Bad
APPETITE FULLNESS / SATISFACTION SWEET CRAVINGS	Following the meal . . . ☐ Feel full, satisfied ☐ Do NOT have sweet cravings ☐ Do NOT desire more food ☐ Do NOT get hungry soon after ☐ Do NOT need to snack before next meal		Following the meal . . . ☐ Feel physically full, but still hungry ☐ Don't feel satisfied; feel like something was missing from meal ☐ Have desire for sweets ☐ Feel hungry again soon after meal ☐ Need to snack between meals
ENERGY LEVELS	Normal energy response to meal: ☐ Energy is restored after eating ☐ Have good, lasting, "normal" sense of energy and well-being		Poor energy response to meal: ☐ Too much or too little energy ☐ Become hyper, jittery, shaky, nervous, or speedy ☐ Feel hyper, but exhausted "underneath" ☐ Energy drop, fatigue, exhaustion, sleepiness, drowsiness, lethargy, or listlessness
MENTAL EMOTIONAL WELL-BEING	Normal qualities: ☐ Improved well-being ☐ Sense of feeling refueled and restored ☐ Upliftment in emotions ☐ Improved clarity and acuity of mind ☐ Normalization of thought processes		Abnormal qualities: ☐ Mentally slow, sluggish, spacey ☐ Inability to think quickly or clearly ☐ Hyper, overly rapid thoughts ☐ Inability to focus/hold attention ☐ Hypo traits: Apathy, depression, sadness ☐ Hyper traits: Anxious, obsessive, fearful, angry, short tempered, or irritable, etc.

Final Words

As you come to the end of your journey through this book, you are faced with many challenges and decision in the near future. Will you stick with the program? Will you be diligent in your exercising? Will you adhere to the metabolic type diet that is best for you? Only you can answer and choose what your path from here will be.

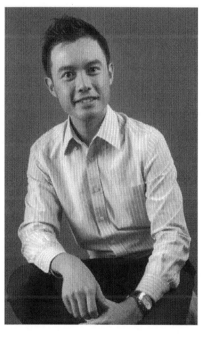

This book has given you the tools and insight you need to make an informed decision about your future health and fitness. I hope I have shown you that a diagnosis of scoliosis does not have to be a death sentence for an active and happy life, that there is something you can do about it, and that you can still take charge of your life and help heal yourself.

No disease has to be a life sentence-your body may be predisposed for certain problems and ailments, but you still possess the power to alter the course you are on and get yourself on the track to a healthier and better way of living.

You have seen how simply finding the right diet and exercise routine can make a world of difference in your pain level and can actually help you have more energy and live a more active life; it can even help to reverse the damage caused by your scoliosis. It is within us, the power to modify how our genes express themselves in us and through us. Genes make us who we are but they do not determine what we are or what we can become. You may suffer from scoliosis, but you are more than the disease.

Starting with one of the most basic human functions- eating- and adding to it a specially developed and tailored exercise program, it is possible to slowly reverse that damage caused by scoliosis. It will not happen overnight and it will not always be easy, but the result is worth it- a better, healthier, and happier you!

I do hope you have enjoyed this book and this accompanying guide that you now have found the tools and inspiration you need to take back control of your life. Even after you have mastered this book to the fullest, the discovery and learning will continue as new and even better discoveries and revelations are made. If you come across any programs, ideas, discoveries, or medical break throughs, feel free to contact me, I would love to hear from you and share our stories.

scoliosis.feedback@gmail.com

If you would like to find out more about other Health In Your Hands products such as other scoliosis books, DVDs, and App go to:

www.HIYH.info

I would be most thankful to you for your suggestions and would happily try to incorporate those in the next edition of this book. Knowledge is power. Use it wisely to promote good health.

Knowledge is power. Use it wisely to promote good health.

Dr Kevin Lau D.C.

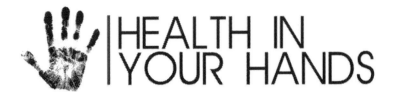

HEALTH IN YOUR HANDS

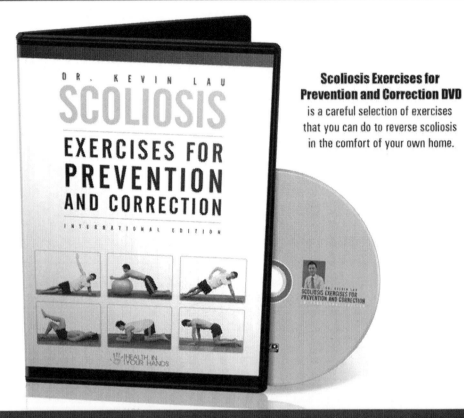

Scoliosis Exercises for Prevention and Correction DVD is a careful selection of exercises that you can do to reverse scoliosis in the comfort of your own home.

For anyone who suffers scoliosis, the main advantages of the DVD are:

- It gives a 60-minute concise expansion of Dr Lau's book by the same name, Health In Your Hands: Your Plan for Natural Scoliosis Prevention and Treatment.
- The Body Balancing section in the DVD explains in detail the correct stretching techniques for scoliosis sufferers to relieve stiffness.
- The Building Your Core section focuses on strengthening the muscles that give stability to your spine. Body Alignment Exercises will improve the overall alignment of your spine.
- All the exercises that feature in the DVD are suitable for pre and post-operative rehabilitation for scoliosis conditions.
- Safe even for those in pain.
- All exercises covered in the Health In Your Hands DVD can be practiced at home, and with no special equipment required.

ScolioTrack

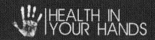
HEALTH IN YOUR HANDS

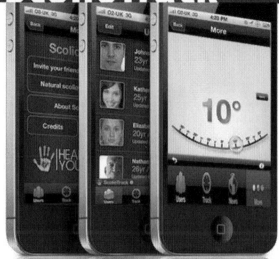

Scoliotrack is a safe and innovative way to track a person's scoliosis condition month to month by using the iPhone accelerometer just as a doctor would with a scoliometer. A scoliometer is an instrument that is used to estimate the amount of curve in a person's spine. It may be used as a tool during screening or as follow-up for scoliosis, a deformity in which the spine curves abnormally.

Features of program

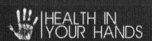

- Can be used with multiple users and saves their data conveniently on the iphone for future checkups

- Tracks and saves a person's Angle of Trunk Rotation (ATR), a key measurement in screening for and planning treatment of scoliosis.

- Tracks a person's height and weight – ideal for growing teenagers with scoliosis or adults who are health conscious.

- Scoliosis progression is graphed making it easy to read month to month changes to a persons scoliosis.

- Displays the latest news feed for scoliosis to keep users informed and up-to-date.

- Full help and easy to follow guides so anyone can track their scoliosis in the comfort of their own home

HEALTH IN YOUR HANDS | Pregnancy Book

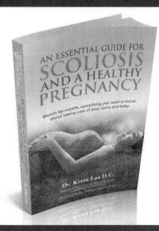

An Essential Guide for Scoliosis and a Healthy Pregnancy: Month-by-month, everything you need to know about taking care of your spine and baby.

COMPLETE, EASY-TO-FOLLOW GUIDE FOR MANAGING YOUR SCOLIOSIS DURING PREGNANCY!

Expert advice to survive pregnancy while suffering from scoliosis. "An Essential Guide for Scoliosis and a Healthy Pregnancy" is a month-by-month guide on covering everything you need to know about taking care of your spine and your baby. The book supports your feelings and empathizes with you throughout your amazing journey towards delivering a healthy baby.

Follow Us

Stay connected with the latest health tips, news and updates from Dr. Lau with the following social media sites. Join the Health In Your Hands page on Facebook to have the opportunity to ask Dr Kevin Lau questions about the book, general questions about their scoliosis, iPhone App called ScolioTrack and Scoliometer or the scoliosis exercise DVD:

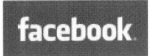 www.facebook.com/HealthInYourHands

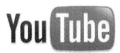 www.youtube.com/DrKevinLau

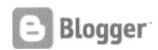 www.DrKevinLau.blogspot.com

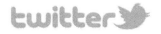 www.twitter.com/DrKevinLau

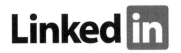 http://sg.linkedin.com/in/DrKevinLau

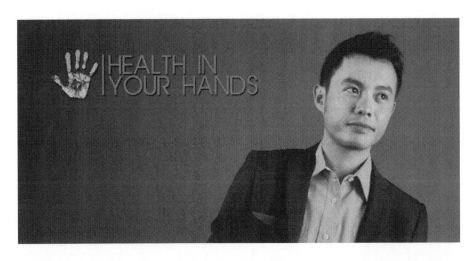

Printed in Great Britain
by Amazon.co.uk, Ltd.,
Marston Gate.